THE NURSE'S DILEMMA

ETHICAL CONSIDERATIONS IN NURSING PRACTICE

Project Director
Barbara L. Tate, R.N., Ed.D.
Dean, College of Nursing
University of Rhode Island
U.S.A.

International Council of Nurses
Florence Nightingale International Foundation
Geneva Switzerland

 Printed in USA by the American Journal of Nursing Company, New York. Price: Swiss francs 9.00, US $3.50 or English £2.50 per copy.

TABLE OF CONTENTS

PREFACE

One of the functions of the Professional Services Committee of the International Council of Nurses is to recommend to the Board of Directors, educational projects to be financed through the income of the Florence Nightingale International Foundation. The Board of Directors at its meeting in March 1975 accepted the PSC recommendation that FNIF funds be used to produce a book based on:

> ". . . the five main facets of the ICN Code for Nurses: Nurses and People, Nurses and Practice, Nurses and Society, Nurses and Co-workers, Nurses and the Profession;
>
> That this publication include a series of contributions by individual nurses on real-life situations in their countries submitted through their member associations;
>
> That this publication be completed for sale at the Congress in Tokyo in 1977. . ."

ICN member associations were asked to disseminate information about this project to nurses and to schools of nursing within their country. Nurses were asked to submit directly to ICN examples of ethical problems they had experienced personally that they did or did not know how to solve. They were told that individuals would not be identified in the publication either by name or country. Nurses from some 25 countries did make submissions.

In some instances individual nurses sent in one or more case studies; in others, a national nurses association sent in a collection of incidents that resulted from group meetings at every level of the association.

Not all of the material received has been published in part because many focused on the same problem, submitting very similar issues although the language, culture and inter-relationships were different.

If there was a commonality throughout the material ICN received, it was that the nurse seemed to feel the matter was her problem alone. The nurse seldom discussed the issue with nursing or medical colleagues. We hope this truly international book on ethical issues — by nurses — for nurses — will help to take away some of that feeling of "aloneness."

We extend our sincere appreciation to each and everyone who in any way contributed to the fulfilment of this ICN/ FNIF project on nursing ethics.

We would like to extend particular thanks to our publisher, the American Journal of Nursing Company, and to the following nurses who formulated the questions following the case studies and generally rounded out the content: from the Faculty of the Department of Nursing, Tel-Aviv University: Rebecca Bergman, Rifka Adams, Lea Greif, Ruth Ron, Aviva Rotenberg; Zeeva Tal from the Ministry of Health, Jerusalem and Olga Weiss, Jerusalem.

Adele Herwitz
Executive Director
International Council of Nurses
and
Honorary Secretary
Florence Nightingale
International Foundation

January 1977

INTRODUCTION

Since its inception the International Council of Nurses has been concerned with both the ethical and the legal aspects of nursing. Although the legal and legislative activities have played a more prominent part in the records of the ICN dating from its origin in 1899, ethical considerations have been uppermost in the minds of many in determining the direction the legislative action would take.

It was not until 1953 that the first code of ethics was finally written and accepted at the Congress in Sao Paulo, Brazil (see p. 73). The code was revised twice, once in 1965 and then, into its present form in 1973 (p. xii).

The ICN Code for Nurses in current use worldwide was adopted at the 1973 Congress in Mexico City. This Code is a broad statement of the nurse's responsibility as a professional person. It touches upon many new areas of nursing responsibility and accountability. This Code, as well as earlier ICN codes of ethics—and indeed, those of all professions—derives from traditional ethical concepts.

It was necessary to look at the responsibility of a professional nurse in today's world and build a code of behaviour which gives general direction adaptable to all cultures. In certain instances advances in medical science have made it possible to make decisions about life and death. The rapid travel and communication throughout the world means that people of a variety of cultures mix together freely in all parts of the world. The dominant group in any area cannot expect all sub-groups to be subjected to its values. Respect of minority group sub-cultures is necessary if mental and physical health of these groups is to be maintained.

The development of nursing as a profession is in various stages in different parts of the world. Progress is closely affiliated with sociological factors within an area or country. The code for nurses at this time includes items which are of ethical derivation but it also includes other items which guide behaviour toward the raising of standards of nurses and nursing.

The 1973 *ICN Code for Nurses* touches on all facets of the life of a nurse as a professional person. It may well vary in interpretation by different individuals and groups. Codes are not law but are guides to all nurses in making critical decisions pertaining to appropriate professional behaviour and actions. A familiarity and study of this universally known code can help us prepare for those unexpected instances when a critical decision must be made immediately and the situation may not appear to have a clear cut right or wrong solution.

A GUIDE FOR THE USE OF THIS BOOK

The purpose of this book is to serve as the basis for discussion among nurses as to what might be appropriate behaviour in the many complex situations they face. Nurses, through their involvement in patient care, are called upon to make many decisions regarding their own behaviour. Situations vary, but certain guidelines for behaviour remain constant. Circumstances may pressure nurses to behave differently at different times. This may or may not be justified, but once the action has been taken, it usually cannot be altered.

The incidents described in this book demonstrate clearly that nursing practice is affected by cultural and religious factors dominant in an area and by the nurse's personal background. Nursing practice is also directly affected by the legislation governing nursing within each country. As a result some things which the nurse is authorized to do in one country may well be illegal in another. Because of laws and customs, some of the situations reported in this book may never occur in some countries. However, with the migration of nurses and other people (potential patients) from one country to another, nurses must be aware of these differences. Nurses are subject to the laws of the country in which they practice. Conversely, nurses do not leave their customs behind as they move, nor do patients and this can lead to conflicts.

This book is an edited compilation of materials submitted by nurses. Many incidents contain the nurses rationale for her action, and/or her own opinion of whether she acted correctly or not. Some leave the judgements entirely to the reader. The editor does not express an opinion of right or wrong interpretation of the Code.

To discuss the full meaning of each of the situations described in this book nurses need to be familiar with the *ICN Code for Nurses* and with the laws of the country in which they are practicing. The Nurse Practice Act is only the basic law from which to start. Many other laws of the country may well affect the decisions a nurse will make under certain circumstances.

The incidents in this book may involve several points of the Code, but central to them all is the fundamental responsibility of the nurse: *to promote health, to prevent illness, to restore health and to alleviate suffering.*

Some of the incidents appear at first to be simple and straight forward. The reader may tend to judge quickly that the nurse's behaviour was "right" or "wrong". However, the more questions the reader asks the more complex the situations appear. A thorough discussion of any one of the incidents will lead the reader to consider many factors which are not obvious upon first reading.

Many of the incidents appear to illustrate poor practice by some colleague on the health team. It is assumed that this is not because poor practice is common, but because an incident of poor practice is remembered vividly.

Other incidents involve actions related to the controversial issues of abortion, euthanasia, and prolongation of life. The book contains many views on these issues, and examples of how some nurses have coped with these problems and how they feel about their own action.

Each incident in the book is followed by some specific questions. In addition, the following questions of a general nature could evoke further discussion of each incident:

1. What portion or portions of the ICN Code for Nurses are applicable in this situation?

2. Do you think the nurse's action was in keeping with the Code?
3. Why do you think she acted as she did?
4. What choices of action were open to the nurse in this situation?
5. If this situation occurred in your work setting, how would you respond?
6. Can you think of a similar incident in your own experience?
7. How did you respond to a similar incident?
8. Was your response to that incident in keeping with the Code?
9. What other choices of action were open to you at that time?
10. Did you think of acting differently in that situation from what you really did do?

INTERNATIONAL COUNCIL OF NURSES
CODE FOR NURSES
ETHICAL CONCEPTS APPLIED TO NURSING
1973

The fundamental responsibility of the nurse is fourfold: to promote health, to prevent illness, to restore health and to alleviate suffering.

The need for nursing is universal. Inherent in nursing is respect for life, dignity and rights of man. It is unrestricted by considerations of nationality, race, creed, colour, age, sex, politics or social status.

Nurses render health services to the individual, the family and the community and coordinate their services with those of related groups.

Nurses and People

The nurse's primary responsibility is to those people who require nursing care.

The nurse, in providing care, promotes an environment in which the values, customs and spiritual beliefs of the individual are respected.

The nurse holds in confidence personal information and uses judgement in sharing this information.

Nurses and Practice

The nurse carries personal responsibility for nursing practice and for maintaining competence by continual learning.

Adopted by the ICN Council of National Representatives, Mexico City in May 1973. All direct quotes in the text are italicized and not otherwise acknowledged.

The nurse maintains the highest standards of nursing care possible within the reality of a specific situation.

The nurse uses judgement in relation to individual competence when accepting and delegating responsibilities.

The nurse when acting in a professional capacity should at all times maintain standards of personal conduct which reflect credit upon the profession.

Nurses and Society

The nurse shares with other citizens the responsibility for initiating and supporting action to meet the health and social needs of the public.

Nurses and Co-Workers

The nurse sustains a cooperative relationship with co-workers in nursing and other fields.

The nurse takes appropriate action to safeguard the individual when his care is endangered by a co-worker or any other person.

Nurses and the Profession

The nurse plays the major role in determining and implementing desirable standards of nursing practice and nursing education.

The nurse is active in developing a core of professional knowledge.

The nurse, acting through the professional organization, participates in establishing and maintaining equitable social and economic working conditions in nursing.

CHAPTER ONE

RESPECT FOR LIFE

The Code for Nurses (1973) states that the nurse should "respect life." This statement replaced "preserved life" in earlier versions. The change was made in the light of modern technology which enables continuation of vital life functions by mechanical means in situations where the irreversible damage would cause immediate death without artificial intervention.

The question of respect for life is deeply rooted in religion, culture and law. There are people of conviction both as proponents and antagonists on this highly charged issue. Each nurse, each patient and in fact, each person holds strong beliefs and feelings about these subjects. Religious teachings, ethnic customs and laws may sometimes conflict. Even each individual may have a different approach to the conflict under different circumstances. Three kinds of situations among others, in which the nurse may be faced with the issue are: life-saving measures for severely malformed infants, heroic measures in irreversible terminal cases and preventing conception or interrupting pregnancy. An additional area which may soon become a reality and a responsibility in nursing is that of decisions regarding bio-engineering.

Nursing is not alone in this quandary. Medicine, law, religion, philosophy and other disciplines are equally troubled. Perhaps the one clear directive that has emerged is that decisions related to respect for life, must be made by a qualified and authorized group and not by a single individual.

A. CONFLICTS RELATED TO MALFORMED INFANTS

Infants are sometimes born with defective bodies and minds. Many times these defects can be seen at birth. Frequently these infants have a very short life span. Sometimes the life span is long, but the quality of life is dependent upon the nature and extent of the deformity as well as the culture in which the person lives. A conflict exists between people as to the appropriate care of these infants. Nurses may make decisions about the care and they may be expected to follow the directions of others. The following examples show a few of the conflicts that can occur.

---

1. ATTITUDES TOWARD DEFORMED CHILDREN

I was working in another country away from my own people. I worked with mothers in labour, delivery and post-partum and with their babies. One day a child was born. A pretty little face but, alas, an ugly spina bifida accompanied with a closed anal sphincter and malformations of the feet. Would it have been better not to allow the infant's first live cry? It was I who uttered the cry I heard within me, "Lord must I put cotton wool in this child's mouth? It would be an act of charity."

Instantaneously the reply came from within me also "Life and death decisions do not belong to me." The newborn child uttered her first cry to which the smile of the mother replied.

The following days were both painful and peaceful. Normally I would not have expected joy but only pain when the mother learned of the many problems. I was astonished to find such a calm mother and one who seemed almost indifferent to the infant's problems and prognosis. The child lived only a few days and the mother showed little grief at her death. Later I learned that it was of prime importance to this mother to have given birth to a living child. To her it meant that the Devil had no hold upon her and she would be able to beget living children.

In later years she did have live and healthy children.

a) What could have been the possible implications of terminating the child's life for the mother? the nurse? others?
b) Do malformations as presented here cause suffering to the child? If so, can this suffering be reduced?
c) What other reactions might the mother have had and how could these affect her future?

---

2. NEWBORN INCOMPATIBLE WITH LIFE

I was working in the labour room one night in a small hospital in a remote area. When the mother had progressed far enough in labour she was transferred to the delivery room. I did not go with her and was not present when her baby was born. Later I went to see her and her baby.

When I asked to see the baby I was told that the baby "was no good" and had been left in a room near the delivery room because it would live but a very short time. The baby did not die in the next hours as expected and so was transferred to a special nursery. The doctor ordered that only water was to be given to the baby as he deemed the baby "incompatible with life." The baby did not live very long but I clearly recall following the order of water only and consequently watching the baby literally starving to death.

I do not recall now the name of the syndrome but I do remember reading about it later in a text. This syndrome was usually fatal early in life but in rare instances children had lived as long as eleven years. The memory of the decision made and my subsequent observations of the baby have remained with me ever since. I still wonder about the decision.

a) Should the family have been consulted?

b) If the nurse was uneasy about the decision what steps should she have taken?

c) What additional information did the nurse need to evaluate the situation (prognosis, other children in family, parent's health, etc.)?

---

3. SEVERELY MALFORMED INFANT

Spina-bifida is an operable condition. Depending on the degree of deformity an operation can be successful and lead to a life which is useful and happy or it can lead to something tragic—a child so grossly damaged and deformed that the quality of life is not acceptable by most standards of humanity. A life sentence of suffering has been passed not only on the child himself but on parents and siblings as well. Today paediatricians are selective. Not all these babies are treated. It is an agonizing decision for them to make.

Parents are asked what they wish done but their knowledge is, of necessity, so limited that they can only do what the doctors seem to advise. Nurses are given the care of a baby who will eventually die, but how soon? One doctor with whom I worked felt that this should be as soon as possible. He said society has denied the child the possibility of meaningful life, and we should not prolong suffering—if, indeed, the child does suffer. He would request that we feed them on water only and give some sedation. Those I nursed were given care and love, and I made a point of doing as much of the care as I could myself. I always hoped parents would not wish to visit, but most did choose to see the baby. I did not encourage handling and I did not talk about feeding. Many of the parents wished their baby to be baptized; a minister or priest was called and we all attended. I gave priority to supporting the parents in their bereavement while the baby lived. I also felt it important to talk to all the younger nurses about the problem and the nursing care, giving them an opportunity to discuss and possibly object. None ever said much, and none objected, but I did not think that all nurses felt able to co-operate in such a course of action.

My own convictions allowed me to cooperate fully with the paediatrician. To me the greatest tragedies of medicine today occur when life is prolonged when it should be allowed to cease. Due to modern science it is possible, for example, to drain the fluid from the head of a hydrocephalic patient when it is obvious that the brain must already be grossly damaged and never likely to recover. This, to me, is an error. If a normal person is unsuccessfully resuscitated, and left handicapped it is unfortunate. However, if that happens we have done our best in good faith and should not reproach ourselves. In the case of a spina-bifida, I believe the matter is quite different.

a) Can the nurse make value judgements about the quality of life of a malformed infant and its family?
b) Who should be partners in the decision of prolonging the life of the malformed infant?
c) What is the responsibility of the experienced nurse to young nurses and students in such traumatic situations?
d) What might the young nurse's silence indicate?
e) What is the responsibility of a supervisor to staff under her supervision?

B. HEROIC EFFORTS

Heroic efforts are often made to sustain life in situations which may offer no hope for recovery and may at the same time prolong suffering for the patient and those near to him.

Discontinuation of heroic efforts—the heart-lung machines, dialysis, intravenous feedings, oxygen, etc. are heart-rending decisions. These actions also have legal implications. Nurses are increasingly faced with these situations.

4. A PATIENT'S WISHES REGARDING RESUSCITATION

The following is the case of Mrs. D., aged 74 years, who was admitted to the coronary care unit with a diagnosis of myocardial infarction. She also had a history of congestive cardiac failure and mitral incompetence.

Shortly after admission the patient had a cardiac arrest; she was successfully resuscitated. She remained on the critical list for some time and progress was slow. She cooperated well with all the treatment and endeared herself to the staff, both nursing and medical, with her courage and delightful sense of humour. Her family, a husband, 3 daughters and 2 sons were very attached to her and she to them. A realist, she was well aware of her serious condition. From a letter she wrote to the family at this time it was obvious that she was satisfied that she had lived a full and happy life and was now quite ready to die.

Mrs. D. continued to make progress and was transferred to the regular medical ward. Here she developed a pleural effusion necessitating frequent chest aspirations. She became progressively weaker and complained of extreme weariness, although one could not help but admire the effort she made to be cheerful.

One morning at 7:30 a.m. she had a cardiac arrest. The team was called and resuscitation was initiated. When I arrived on the scene the relatives were gathered outside the room, all very distraught. Mrs. D. was transferred to the coronary care unit but never regained consciousness and was pronounced dead at 12:25 p.m.

This incident raises some interesting and complex questions. I personally feel that there should be a greater appreciation for team decisions and that nurses should be more vocal in the management of such patients. It is usually the nurse with whom the patients have had the most conversation and expressed their feelings about their illness and their prognosis.

a) Was the second resuscitation warranted?
b) Should decisions of this kind be taken in advance, since the actual situation leaves no time for deliberation?
c) Should decisions be taken about each patient individually, or in accordance with some broad generalization about age or medical condition?
d) Is the criterion the benefit of the patient, allowing the word "benefit" to mean more than the prolongation of life?
e) How can the nurse preserve the integrity of the patient keeping in mind her own approach to death?
f) In what way can the team alleviate the distress of the relatives?
g) Should the team involve the family in reaching a decision? If so, how?

5. TURNING OFF THE MACHINE

I work in an 8-bed intensive care unit of a rehabilitation hospital. All the beds are occupied by severely disabled patients. One of these is a 20-year old girl who was in a car accident a year ago. She suffered severe head injuries and never regained consciousness. Her vital signs are kept at a normal level by machines.

The girl's family visit her regularly. The mother resigned from her job to be near her daughter most of the day. Two young brothers are left to their own resources much of the time. The father works at two jobs to meet family expenses.

During her stay with us, several attempts were made to retain life with reduced or discontinued heroic effort but collapse followed immediately.

The chief doctor called a meeting of all senior staff on the ward, including myself, to discuss the situation. Several suggestions came up, among others to disconnect the machines. To this, different reactions were taken by the participants and no agreement could be reached. No action was taken.

a) What arguments might the team members have put forward?

b) In view of the differences of opinion, how could a decision be reached?

c) What is the place of the family in making a decision?

C. CONTRACEPTION AND/OR INTERRUPTION OF PREGNANCY

Many philosophical and scientific questions influence the nurse's belief and behaviour on this issue. Laws sometimes conflict with belief and sometimes call for interpretations of terms. When is a foetus alive? Under the circumstances may continuation of pregnancy constitute a threat to the life of the mother? What are the implications of pregnancy resulting from rape or incest? Should decisions regarding pregnancy be different for minors, the subnormal, and the mentally ill? Should pregnancies with high-risk abnormality of the infant be continued? To what degree might social psychological and economic problems influence such decisions?

6. A REQUEST FOR STERILIZATION

I am working in a family planning centre with a young couple as clients. It is the second marriage for them both. She has a 6-year old daughter from her previous marriage. They now have a new baby girl. She is quite adamant that she wants no more babies. She has insisted that her husband have a vasectomy.

The father of the young man has asked me to intervene and convince them that his daughter-in-law should be the one who is sterilized. The young man's father objects to the vasectomy because there are no sons to carry on the man's family name. His rationale also includes: the marriage thus far has been through considerable difficulty and he is doubtful that it will continue; the young wife is emotionally unstable and, since she is not a good mother, she should be sterilized.

Although I have made observations which make me tend to agree with the man, I certainly cannot make these kinds of decisions for my clients. I informed the man I could not interfere and suggested that he talk with his son. If his son wishes to listen to the council of his father, he could. If the son had questions I, as a family planning staff member could answer, I would. I made it very clear that I could not make the decision for them. It must be a mutual decision between man and wife.

Through his interference, the father has delayed the final decision regarding the sterilization. The young couple are currently successful in the use of other contraceptive techniques.

a) What aspects should be weighed before concurring with a patient's request for sterilization?
b) Are there circumstances in which nurses should recommend sterilization?
c) What resources can the nurse use in helping couples prevent pregnancy?
d) What other action might the nurse take in meeting the health needs of this couple?
e) In what way could the nurse help other family members concerned with the problem?

---

7. CLINIC FOR TERMINATION OF PREGNANCY

As a nurse, I have a respect for life. To me abortion is not compatible with a respect for life. I am currently working in a clinic where pregnancies are terminated. As a part of my work I prepare all the material needed for the intervention.

I assist the doctor who uses this material in the operating

theatre. If the pregnancy is beyond 12 or 14 weeks in duration the technique is different, but I must still carry out the preparation, assist with the procedure and help with the expulsion of the foetus.

I do take care of the patient and see to her needs. At the same time, I must also care for the foetus, sometimes seeing it live briefly and die, weigh it, measure it, and forward it. All these activities call for me to contribute actively, on medical order, to suppress human life, to destroy a life unable to defend itself. This is in contradiction with my conscience. It is not acting according to the respect for life which I feel so strongly.

I am not the only one who feels this conflict. For me, there is only one action I can take. I must change my place of work. My feelings tell me that for nurses this is not a real solution to the dilemma.

a) Should a nurse take employment in any agency where the philosophy and content of the services are not in accord with her beliefs?
b) To whom could this nurse have turned for guidance and support?
c) Does resigning from the position contribute to the solution of the problem?
d) Were there alternatives to resigning?

---

8. TEACHING STUDENTS CONTRACEPTION AND ABORTION

I am working in a college health service in a coeducational Catholic college. The question frequently arises as to what advice and counsel to give a college student when she requests information and advice about birth control or asks questions pertaining to her newly discovered pregnant state. Knowing that the college functions under the Roman Catholic doctrine, which discourages dissemination of information on birth control and prohibits abortion, what is the college health nurse to do? In most cases I have proceeded with careful individual counselling offering several alternatives and allowing the student to reach her own decision for action. When she was unable to come to any decision, I arranged an appointment at a family planning centre, abortion counselling service or a right to life centre. She could keep the appointment or not, which ever she chose to do.

As the college health nurse at this particular institution I have no open option to use my own sound judgement in order to help this bewildered individual sort out her future. If I am known to adapt to a belief of the patient which conflicts with a belief of the church, I could not continue in my position and students would be deprived of what I consider to be their rightful care.

A further complicating issue is, what is the department of nursing authorized to teach with regard to family planning when developing its curriculum in obstetrical nursing? I know that in my experience here a comprehensive text on family planning was recommended to the nursing students and we were all told we would be responsible for reading and learning this information but it would not be discussed in class. A letter from "some concerned parents" was sent to the president of the college requesting/demanding that the nursing faculty be hired not only for their academic qualifications, but for their ideological philosophy and adherence to the teaching of the church.

a) Are there circumstances which would justify the decision of a school to limit curriculum in a way that may later deprive patients of their rightful care?
b) Can students learn to help the patient if they do not have clinical experience or theoretical content related to all facets of reproduction?
c) What measures might a nurse educator take in order to influence a policy of the school with which she disagrees?

d) How might a nurse educator act when instructed by her employer to omit course content that her students might later need to know?

e) What are the possible implications of exposing students to a text book without further discussion and feedback?

---

9. A DISAPPOINTED MIDWIFERY STUDENT

In my country approximately 1200 student nurses qualify for the General Register each year. Many of these take midwifery post-basic courses as soon as possible after registration. As there are not sufficient places in our midwifery schools many Registered General Nurses, in preference to waiting for two to three years for midwifery training at home, go to another country. I was one of the many impatient nurses anxious to have Midwifery and in September 1974 I started Midwifery Training in another country.

Following two weeks of theoretical instruction students were assigned to various clinical areas. I was assigned to the Labour ward (Delivery suite) and spent two weeks there. At first I did not ask too many questions but carried out the duties assigned to me. I did become aware that I was giving "an injection" once a day to a number of women. I became suspicious and asked what the aim of the therapy was. I was told that this would be explained to me later. This made me more suspicious, so mustering all my courage I asked for an immediate explanation. The explanation I got was "it is sterilizing the patient for one year from that date." I then refused to give any further injections. Shortly after this I was assigned to the Antenatal ward which had a four-bed room for women who were to have a therapeutic abortion. In this case I refused to have anything to do with the ladies confined to this area. On one occasion I refused to accompany back from the operating theatre a woman who had had a therapeutic abortion. The strain of constantly saying "no" was beginning to affect me. I talked with some of the staff hoping they would see the problem of therapeutic abortion as I did—the killing of an innocent human being. Some were sympathetic, others skeptical and a few I felt were inclined to come round to my point of view. I knew that during my midwifery training I would spend some time in the operating theatre where I would be expected to assist at such procedures so I approached the Matron of the hospital to explain that I had various problems on ethical grounds. To my amazement, she asked why I bothered to come there to do my midwifery training. I did try to explain that I could never consider that therapeutic abortion or sterilization were part of midwifery for me. It was I felt to no avail.

Rather than continue in these sad circumstances I packed my bags and returned home the next day. I was a disappointed midwifery student but happy that I had taken the correct action.

a) How can the school ensure that the philosophy, theoretical content and clinical experience of their program is known and understood by the candidates?
b) Do students have a right to request a change of program?
c) Can schools adapt their programs in accordance with the beliefs of individual students?
d) Should the nurse have come to a country to study knowing of the legal and cultural differences which she could not accept?
e) Is family planning and interruption of pregnancy a legitimate component of midwifery training?

CHAPTER TWO

NURSES AND PEOPLE

A. VALUES, CUSTOMS AND BELIEFS

The Code for Nurses states that *the nurse, in providing care, promotes an environment in which the values, customs and spiritual beliefs of the individual are respected.*

Care may meet the individual's biological needs, be a therapeutic (medical) regime, provide emotional support and/or consist of health education. The environment includes any such physical setting of the individual as: his home, school, place of work, health center, clinic, custodial center or hospital. It also includes the psycho-social atmosphere, such as interpersonal relationships, behavioural norms, socialization process, and so on.

The nurse cannot control or direct the total environment, but the nurse has a major role in utilizing available resources and in planning for or developing resources not immediately available.

Most important is the fact that the nurse is the care giver who has the most extensive contact with the individual and his family. It is the nurse who is best able to assess the operating values, customs, and beliefs and incorporate her knowledge of them in directing the nursing care and the care of other therapists.

Recognition and respect of the values, customs and beliefs of the individual does not always mean actively accepting them if so doing may impede a patient's recovery or endanger his life. One patient's (or relative's) beliefs may cause harm or discomfort to another. Some customs or values may conflict with the nurse's basic beliefs or values and the nurse may not in good conscience be able to comply with them. Such situations set up ethical problems for the nurse.

10. OBSERVING RELIGIOUS DIETARY LAWS

I was working in an Eastern country and over a period of time I cared for a number of diabetic patients. Many of these patients were devout religious peoples and observed their dictary laws very rigidly. It was not too difficult to work out a diet which was appropriate for patients of Muslim, Jewish or Hindu faiths.

However, there was always a conflict in my mind while caring for these patients. The only insulin available some times was made from the pancreas of an animal that was forbidden to the faithful followers. Occasionally bovine insulin was not available or produced an allergic reaction. It was necessary to use that made from the pig for a Jewish or Muslim patient. Occasionally that made from the pig was not available and only bovine could be used for Hindu patients.

a) In your country with its specific ethnic and religious backgrounds, how would this type of problem affect your functions?
b) What are the factors to be considered when faced with a decision of informing or not informing a patient about medication or dietary sources?
c) With whom can the nurse discuss such problems?
d) If the order is in conflict with patient's wishes, what are the alternatives for treatment?
e) Does the nurse have a responsibility to know the patient's beliefs?
f) What is the nurse's responsibility for compatibility between treatment and belief?

11. LIFE-SAVING MEASURES VERSUS RELIGIOUS BELIEFS

In 1970, I was in charge of a 360-bed district hospital up country in a remote area in Africa. Although we had physical facilities equipped for ten midwives to take care of our 25-bed maternity ward, lack of midwives brought about a situation where we were reduced to one midwife for the entire unit. When this midwife went away on leave I had to conduct deliveries in addition to carrying the general administration of the entire hospital.

One morning, a woman in labour was admitted to the delivery ward. On examination I found her to have a twin pregnancy. She had not been attending the prenatal clinic and looked to me to be clinically anaemic. Blood was taken for haemoglobin, grouping and crossmatching in preparation for transfusing her.

The haemoglobin was estimated at 4.7 grammes per cent. It was decided that she should be transfused with four pints of blood. I explained the situation to the patient and told her why she needed the blood. The patient told me she was a "Jehovah's Witness" and therefore could not consent to a transfusion. I sent for the husband with the hope of eliciting his support and understanding. The husband agreed with the wife. They would not consent.

A litre of dextrose in saline was put up to keep the vein open. Fifteen minutes later the first twin was born and he was in good condition. Although there was very little bleeding, the patient collapsed and at this stage I was faced with having to restore her to a better state of health. I called a doctor who felt that nothing much could be done except transfusing her which he was not prepared to do without the patient's consent.

I felt that to save the life of the unborn twin something had to be done. I discussed my feelings with the doctor. He had no objection to my taking the responsibility for giving her a transfusion. The transfusion was started under complete cover with no relatives allowed in the room and the patient unconscious. During the second pint of the transfusion, the patient regained consciousness and protested the treatment. The intravenous fluid was changed back to dextrose in saline. The second baby was born shortly after the blood transfusion had been discontinued. He was in good condition. The bleeding was minimal, but again the mother collapsed. More blood was given intravenously with a view to resuscitating her. It was considered a life-saving measure. This time the response was poor. Although she had all of the four pints of blood crossmatched for her, she never recovered consciousness and died four hours later.

While the Code for Nurses served to guide me in the promotion and restoration of the patient's health, this was contradicted by the need to respect the spiritual belief of the patient. In these circumstances, I found my conscience the surest guide; I did all I could to save the life of the patient. I feel I did save the life of the second baby.

a) Under what circumstances would life-saving measures be put ahead of religious beliefs?
b) Is there a difference in the impact of the conflict when the nurse is alone in such a situation, and when she is in a larger medical center and can consult with others?
c) Were there alternatives to the therapeutic care given by this nurse?
d) What are the legal aspects of this case? Do guidelines exist in your country?
e) Is there a difference between obtaining consent for potential or for actual life-saving situations?

---

12. PATIENT'S DISCRIMINATION AGAINST A STUDENT

I am a European and a prepared nurse instructor who was working in a country of another culture. I experienced hearing a patient request that a student nurse from a minority group of that country should not be allowed to touch him. The student nurse was a good student whom I knew was giving good knowledgeable care to patients and was also kind, gentle and tactful with patients. The refusal of this patient to accept care given by the student was based solely upon his feelings pertaining to the ethnic minority group she represented.

I had a discussion with this patient in an attempt to influence his decision, but it appeared to arouse anxiety. In the interest of the patient's welfare, I felt I should change the assignment for this student and I gave the nursing care to the patient myself. I used the period of time I spent with the patient to discuss his interracial feelings with the goal of helping the patient accept the student nurse as a competent learner capable of giving him care.

a) Should the nurse instructor have discussed this with the patient?
b) Is the bedside an appropriate place to try to change attitudes?
c) How could the student be taught to give non-discriminatory care and still accept the patient's right to discriminate?
d) What would you have done in such a situation?
e) Are there circumstances where you accept the patient's right to discriminate?

---

13. CONFLICTS WITH RELIGIOUS BELIEFS

A woman of Roman Catholic faith was discharged from the clinic after giving birth to her eighth child. The public health nurse was asked to go into the home to follow the progress of the mother and infant for the first few weeks. In talking with her the nurse learned that the mother was quite anxious not to have any more children.

During her visits the nurse informed the patient of the family planning clinics available to her. She also discussed the various contraceptive measures from which she could select the one she felt the most appropriate to her needs.

Subsequently, the patient visited her physician, also a Roman Catholic, and told him of her discussion with the nurse. The physician immediately called the nurse and her supervisor and advised them to cease any such discussion with his patients. He said it was not the nurses' business to discuss family planning with any patients and particularly not if the patient was of the Roman Catholic faith.

a) In your country what is the nurse's responsibility regarding response to a patient's questions which are in conflict with the principles of her religion?
b) To whom is the nurse primarily responsible?
c) What are some of the considerations that would influence the nurse's behaviour in this situation?
d) How does the policy of the health agency or service influence the nurse's decision?

B. PERSONAL INFORMATION HELD IN CONFIDENCE

The Code for Nurses states that: *The nurse holds in confidence personal information and uses judgement in sharing this information.* Nursing is a health service in which virtually all decisions are made for the welfare of the patient.

Part of the nursing process is to encourage the patient to express himself freely, and to share his problems and feelings with the nurse.

Patients under stress frequently reveal thoughts and ideas which they ordinarily would not want others to know. Later, they may regret or even fear having made such confidences. Sometimes, these revelations may relate directly to the illness or affect the recovery process; sometimes they may have an indirect effect on the patient or others within the patient's circle of family, friends or associates. The nurse may thus have information he or she feels should be passed on to others.

Sometimes these confidential comments relate to the illness; sometimes not. The following illustrate experiences where different nurses have used their judgement to determine when to share information.

---

14. A PATIENT'S DEPRESSION

A nurse was caring for a patient who was being treated for a back injury. The treatment was conservative and surgery had not been suggested. The treatment was carried out for many days and included physical therapy. The progress was slow. The pain returned regularly and the increase in activity was very slow.

This once energetic and hard-working man became very depressed by what he saw as the progress or lack of it. He did not have the patience to continue the treatment. He felt at best his physical activity would be limited compared to that to which he was accustomed.

During a conversation with the nurse, he mentioned he was contemplating suicide. This was the only solution he could see to his problem. As soon as he had voiced this plan, he immediately asked the nurse to be absolutely silent and not tell anyone of his thoughts.

The nurse cared for him the rest of that day with every sense alert to the possibility he would attempt suicide. She took every precaution possible short of sitting with the patient constantly. At the end of the day, however, she felt she must break the patient's request for silence. She reported to the nurses on the next shift and to the physician, the patient's statements. Everyone was alerted to protect the patient and to help him learn to cope with this problem without actually informing the patient of the breach of confidence.

The patient appeared to be improved physically and mentally when he was discharged from the hospital.

a) What should the nurse say to the patient's request for silence?

b) What should the nurse say, if anything, to her colleagues?
c) Does it make a difference if the nurse is asked not to reveal a confidence before the confidence is given? After it is given?
d) Should confidential information be entered on the patient's records? If so, under what circumstances, and in what form?

---

15. MEDICAL HISTORY TOLD IN CONFIDENCE

A young unmarried woman was admitted to the hospital with excessive uterine bleeding, which she explained was connected with her monthly period. She stated that this had occurred several times over the course of the past year and was of great concern to her.

A student nurse, of the approximate age of the patient, was caring for her the day after admission. The patient told the student that she was certain she was pregnant and had taken some medications which she had been told would bring about an abortion. She did not want anyone even the doctor, to know about this. She asked the student nurse not to tell anyone, particularly the doctor.

The student nurse knew she should not reveal information given by the patient in confidence. However, she felt the proper treatment for the patient could not be carried out unless the doctor knew all the related facts of the patient's history. The student told the entire story to the doctor. The doctor then proceeded to talk with the patient phrasing his questions in such a way that the patient eventually told the doctor the same information herself. The doctor was then able to prescribe the appropriate treatment and still not reveal the breach of confidence.

a) What might have been the impact on the patient if the information was not disclosed?

b) Are there any circumstances which justify keeping medical history confidential?
c) What might have resulted if the patient knew of the breach of confidence?

---

16. LONG-TERM MEDICAL RECORDS

As a school nurse, I am faced with the ethical problem of protection of information about the pupils. Accurate records about the pupils help the nurses maintain good care for pupils over a long period of time. The health records for each student accompany him from kindergarten on through his entire educational experience. If he changes residence and/or schools his record is transferred with him.

The record contains information of the state of his health at regular intervals. It builds a continuous record of his physical and psychological development. It also contains information which pertains to family life and environmental factors which may influence his health and be pertinent in giving health care. The rationale for keeping this complete a record is clearly for the student's benefit. It provides for continuity and follow-up in care and treatment; it records successive treatments and observations for evaluation of progress; it passes on needed information to health personnel when there is a change in the individuals responsible for the students' health.

The ethical problem occurs when particular accounts which once seemed essential for helping the student, remain in the record over a long period of years. The record may leave a mark that will accompany the student for many years. It might well change the attitude of someone toward him and even insult or injure him in his later relationships. Medical records should not be able to leave such a mark on a child for a long time.

Some examples of problems from records are:

A boy was sent to the mental health clinic because of many adolescent problems. Because of this note in his record, he was not accepted in the army with those from his particular age group. Many discussions ensued and at a later time he was allowed to serve as a regular soldier and had no difficulty in fulfilling his responsibilities.

A 6-year old girl hospitalized after her father attempted to have intercourse with her. Her father was later hospitalized. The details of this episode which were essential to her care at the time remained in her record in the schools and accompanied her for many years.

The mother of this pupil is a prostitute. The pupil has a brother and a sister both of whom have unknown fathers.

It is possible in all these instances that the mental trauma to the child will cause a problem in the future. The information might be of use in treating later illnesses. However, the initial treatment may have alleviated the problem for all time and his development will continue normally. Questions asked by later health personnel with access to these records might be the only way that these incidents would later disturb an otherwise normal adjustment to life.

a) What is the impact on the student when these records are perused by each health professional who later contacts this student for any reason?
b) How can we assure they would always be used with complete professional confidence?
c) How could special archives be developed where only limited personnel had access to the material and allowed it to be used only in case of documented need?

17. CONFESSION OF A CRIME

Many years ago a member of the government was assassinated in the centre of the capital city. Several people were arrested; one of them was injured and he was taken to the hospital. The police were investigating the case. The injured man was examined by the police but in the end it was concluded by them that he was innocent. Nothing was proved to be against him.

However, he showed many signs of anxiety and after some days he called the night nurse. He confessed to her that he was the one who had murdered the member of the government. The nurse assured him that she would not tell anyone about it but she strongly advised him to confess to the priest of the hospital. He eventually did so. Two people now knew the important secret but neither felt they could tell the police about it. Both of them felt they were tied to secrecy by their professional obligation to the patient. The priest visited the patient quite often.

a) How should the nurse respond when the patient asks for a promise of confidentiality?
b) What is the responsibility of the nurse as a citizen?
c) Does the fact that another person is also in the patient's confidence influence the nurse's responsibility for whatever action she takes?
d) If a conflict of conscience arises, is the nurse's primary responsibility to the patient or to others who are involved or endangered?

C. INFORMING THE PATIENT

Inherent in nursing is respect for —— the rights of man.

One of the rights of man is the right to knowledge about himself. In the case of a patient knowledge of a diagnosis, the treatment, the prognosis or other facts may help or hinder in his care. Both the physician and the nurse are in a position to give or withhold information. Such information may be requested by the patient or his family; sometimes, information is related voluntarily by those giving care. Laws of some countries regulate decisions on this subject; customs in different cultures vary on this subject. The following illustrations are examples of conflicts pertaining to this right of man to know.

---

18. WITHHOLDING KNOWLEDGE OF STERILIZATION

The setting is in a rural mountain community. A family of ten lives in a cramped and tumble-down two room house. The building is badly in need of repair.

The father, Mr. S. is 39 years old, obese, unshaven and unemployed. He went to the third grade in school and stopped because he had "better things to do," worked in the coal mines once but stopped when his heart started to "give out." He now works an occasional odd job.

The mother is pale, small boned, and 27 years old. Looking at her, one can see that she was pretty when younger but eight childbirths in close succession, and the work of raising a large family have taken their toll. She is eight months pregnant with their ninth child.

The children range in age from 11 months to 12 years. There are no twins although three boys were born within a 28-month period. Their mother almost died during the second and third of those pregnancies.

Through the years, Mr. S. has developed a large appetite for alcohol. He is out most of the time and often comes in late at night after drinking for hours. When he is drunk, he is mean. It seems he vents anger at his life situation and this anger flairs out at his wife and children. For the past several years sexual intercourse between father and mother could easily be described as rape. The mother would never leave him; it is against her nature to leave her man.

She is a "good" mother, conscientious about keeping the

children immunized at the local clinic, and openly turns to health professionals for guidance. She usually follows medical advice closely. When the last baby was born, a year ago, she was strongly urged to use some form of birth control. She was in favour of this, but the husband was vehemently against it. This man, ineffective even in the rural mountain society, held tightly to his procreative abilities.

During this pregnancy she has been continually at risk. She was anaemic at the start, she had at least three bladder infections and one episode of pyelonephritis. She refused hospitalization because her husband was drinking heavily and she feared for her children if they were left alone with him. During her ninth month, with close supervision by the county nurses, she seemed to be in relatively fair condition.

When she entered labour, her husband found a neighbor to take them to the hospital forty miles away. Once in the hospital she progressed well, dilating steadily to seven centimetres. At this point she stopped; the contractions were ineffective and after one hour the condition was obviously maternal dystocia. The baby's heart-beat was decreasing. The decision for a caesarean section to save the mother and child was made. The husband was not available to sign the operative permit, although the mother timidly signed it.

The baby was delivered safely; but after delivery the uterus ruptured. Quickly a decision was made to perform a complete hysterectomy allowing one ovary to remain. Following the operation, the mother stabilized and within two weeks she was home again with the healthy new baby.

The obstetrician and the maternity nurses were familiar with this woman's social background. They made the decision not to tell her or her husband that the sterilizing procedure had been performed. This decision was based on fears of how the husband would react if he knew he had lost his ability for social notoriety: having a large family. There was a very real fear that this man would physically abuse the newborn, even more than he had his other offspring. The fears were increased by the fact he might view the child as the cause of his wife's infertility.

The information was kept secret from the husband. When Mrs. S's menstrual periods ceased, she asked the county nurse why and was told of the decision to perform the life preserving procedure. Apparently she accepted her condition with a certain amount of relief and she too keeps the information from her husband. The story of the childbirth is passed on to new health professionals on the case as background information. As far as we know, the family situation exists as before with alcohol and poverty working in a vicious cycle but the husband is unaware that his wife can have no more children.

a) Does the team have the right to withhold information from the wife or the husband? If so, under what circumstances?
b) Was the timing of informing the woman of the extensive nature of her surgery important? Why?
c) What factors should be considered if a decision is made to inform the husband about the surgery? Who should be consulted? Are there resources and persons available who could lessen the negative aspects of the husband's receiving this information?

---

19. DIAGNOSIS INFLUENCING COOPERATION

A patient was admitted to the hospital for diagnostic procedures for a chest ailment. He had been suffering chest pains, shortness of breath and increasing fatigue for some time. Many tests were performed and the patient was given medications and treatment for emphysema. However, the physician had not discussed the diagnosis, treatment or prognosis with the patient.

The patient kept asking the staff nurse for information. She felt reluctant to discuss the matter with the patient until the physician had at least outlined the essential items. The nurse normally expected to help the patient learn about his illness but not until after the physician had disclosed the diagnosis.

As the days continued the physician did not respond precisely to the patient's questions. Neither did the physician respond to the nurse's suggestions that the patient be informed.

One day when the patient refused the medications and treatments, the nurse told the patient his diagnosis. She then proceeded to discuss the prognosis if the treatment regimen was followed carefully and the prognosis if he did not continue the treatment as ordered.

The patient again was cooperative with the nurse when she treated him. However, the physician severely reprimanded the nurse for her forwardness in assuming what, he said, was the physician's rightful role. He felt the patient should not have known his diagnosis or his prognosis. The nurse felt she was justified in telling him. He had a right to know. His care required his cooperation if he was to have any relief.

a) How should the nurse respond when asked by the doctor not to answer the patient's questions?
b) Can a nurse teach a patient to help himself when he knows nothing about his illness? If so, how can she implement the teaching?
c) When a patient asks for information about his illness and is not answered, what reactions can the nurse expect? How will these affect her care?
d) What information should the nurse gather and consider before deciding whether to tell the patient his diagnosis and/or prognosis?
e) What persons should take the responsibility of telling or not telling the patient his diagnosis?

20. INFORMING PATIENTS

A post-basic student was caring for a 77-year old man who had a colostomy. The colostomy was necessary because of an extensive malignant growth. The patient was not told of the malignancy nor that the colostomy must remain as long as the patient lived.

In the country where the student was studying, patients are virtually never told of diagnoses when there is little or no hope of complete cure. They are sometimes told a diagnosis they recognize as readily curable.

The student was in great conflict about this. He learned that the patient was moderately wealthy, had made no will, and had numerous business decisions awaiting him when he was well and returned to work. Following local custom, the student did not speak of the nature of the patient's illness with him. The student was very upset when the patient died without having had the opportunity to put his business affairs in order.

a) Were there alternatives for the nurse to help the patient settle his affairs without telling him his diagnosis?
b) How might a nurse react when his or her beliefs are in conflict with the policies of the agency employing him or her? In what way, if any, does the post-basic student differ from an employee in this situation?
c) Should the nurse volunteer information about a diagnosis or prognosis to a patient who does not indicate a wish to be told?
d) How can nurse educators and administrators help guide nurses in making such crucial decisions objectively?

21. WITHHOLDING A DIAGNOSIS

Cheryl was a student nurse who entered the General Programme in 1972. Some months after she entered the programme and after several attacks of tonsillitis, Cheryl was diagnosed as having acute lymphatic leukaemia. Her parents were told of the situation and were specifically requested by the consultant as was the entire nursing staff, not to divulge the diagnosis to Cheryl.

Owing to her illness Cheryl quickly dropped behind in her class. Recognizing that the hospital environment was not in the best interest of her precarious health, employment outside the hospital was suggested. After she entered her first remission, she found a position she liked as a secretary in a commercial enterprise.

Cheryl maintained reasonable health under a specific anti-mitotic regime. At approximately 5- to 6-month intervals, she required one or two days of hospitalization to have the blood content and volume restored to normal limits. On each occasion for the first two years, she greeted the staff warmly and seemed to enjoy the break in her usual routine of living that hospital treatment required.

During the third year of her illness Cheryl's attitude to the staff altered considerably and the staff found it increasingly uncomfortable to be in her presence. She rarely asked questions and withdrew from any social interaction. The periods of hospitalization altered gradually so that, three years after the diagnosis was established, Cheryl was admitted with a large necrosing area extending from the perineum into the buttock and enlarging rapidly.

The consultant caring for Cheryl maintained a rigorous system for infection control of his hospitalized leukaemic patients. They were segregated in single rooms and neither staff nor visitors were allowed into the rooms without paper caps, gowns, masks and overshoes.

As Cheryl passed into the terminal phase of her illness, the nursing staff asked repeatedly for the medical staff to discuss with her her ultimate prognosis. Had this been done, it was believed that the charade of possible recovery would have been dropped between Cheryl and her family allowing them at least the possibility of open expression. A few days before her death Bromptons Cocktail was commenced but at the same time to the amazement of the nursing staff the rigorous isolation of the patient was continued despite entreaties from the nursing staff.

I think in retrospect the situation angered us. We believed that the closeness of other human beings to Cheryl particularly in the last phase of her tragic illness would have been an expression of our very humaneness. We were angry I believe at ourselves because we had obeyed instructions and lived a lie. Perhaps being less than open with Cheryl was easier for us than making a case to the consultant for her release from her world of loneliness and deprivation. The final indignity was the introduction of Bromptons without any cessation in the standards of protective isolation and while the case for freedom from isolation was still being considered, Cheryl died.

a) Are there other aspects to living which enrich human experience and which are almost as important as life itself?
b) What may have caused Cheryl to withdraw and what could the nurses have done to help her?
c) What support could the nurses have offered Cheryl to express her feelings?
d) What was the nurses' responsibility to Cheryl's mother and how could they have helped her?

---

22. PROTECTING AN ACCIDENT VICTIM

Recently, whilst working on evening duty in a small country hospital as Sister-in-charge, the victims of a road accident were admitted to my ward. The driver of the vehicle which had left the road and overturned spilling the children out, was the children's mother. She and her four children had all been personally known to me for some time.

One child died shortly after admission. The two middle children, both boys, were nearly scalped, but had their scalp flaps sutured in place and made uneventful recoveries. The smallest daughter eventually completely lost the use of one arm. The eldest child, a girl of thirteen, suffered severe head injuries and died shortly after admission. The mother suffered contusions and abrasions, however, the greatest area of concern was her hysterical mental state in regard to the injuries to her children when she was driving the car.

Despite tranquillizers, this mental condition did not improve until she was heavily sedated later in the night. Throughout the evening her greatest concern was for her eldest daughter who had apparently been the quietest at the scene of the accident and whom she instinctively felt was in the most danger.

Because of my position on the ward and the fact that I was personally known to her, she constantly entreated me to inform her of the childrens' condition. When it became obvious that the daughter was about to die, I asked the doctor what I should tell the mother as he was busy in the operating theatre and could not speak to her himself.

The woman's husband lived some distance away and could not be contacted for several hours, and I was instructed that, because of her distress, the doctor would prefer to inform her in the company of her husband, and until that time I was to re-assure her at all costs.

Over the next few hours, during my ministrations to her, she repeatedly queried me about the children and particularly the eldest daughter. It went strongly against my conscience to have to look her in the eye and repeat a lie of such magnitude.

She was finally sedated and early next morning when her husband and doctor told her the real news her distress was heralded with the cry "Why did she lie to me?"

Through various circumstances, I have not seen her since but her husband told me that, although she understood my instructions had come from her doctor, she felt my behaviour and his had amounted to unethical interference. She no longer considers me a friend. Try as I will, I cannot believe that my action in this case was ethical.

a) Did the medical team participate in conduct that could be called ethical in the belief it would justify the patient's well-being, or did they overstep the bounds of reasonable interference?
b) If the charge nurse, in trying to follow the procedure indicated by the doctor, felt she was transgressing strongly against her conscience, what should she do?
c) Under what circumstances, if any, would you believe it ethical to withhold the truth from a patient?
d) Would it help the nurse if she understood the reasons for the mother's rejection and blame? How could she use such knowledge to help the mother and herself?
e) What were the possible dangers or advantages of temporarily withholding the information of the child's death? How could this knowledge influence the nurse's action?
f) Was the fact that the nurse was a friend of the woman a deciding factor in this case?

---

23. A SURGICAL ACCIDENT

A student nurse was assisting in the operating theatre. She had scrubbed and was passing instruments for a partial gastrectomy on a 45-year old female patient. During the course of the surgery, the scalpel being used to excise the stomach tissue slipped and a large gash resulted in the spleen. Because of this, it was necessary to remove the spleen immediately.

Further on during the same operation, the clamp that was holding the bowel near the lower portion of the stomach was also clamping off the head of the pancreas. This circumstance was of such duration that approximately one-third of the pancreas needed to be removed before final closure of the incision.

The student later learned that the patient had never been advised of the removal of other organs than the original portion of the stomach. The student is concerned as to her responsibility.

a) If the student is convinced that a patient should have certain information which may not reach him from other sources (and which may have legal implications) what avenues are available to her?
b) If the student keeps silent, does she become an accomplice to the damage?
c) Is there a legal rather than ethical responsibility in such a case?
d) If this is basically a problem of medical ethics, does it implicate the student? If so, how?

---

24. WITHHOLDING KNOWLEDGE OF AVAILABLE SERVICES

A nurse caring for pre-natal patients in a clinic was working with a patient in the fourth month of pregnancy. At this time the patient learned of the possible effects of rubella upon an unborn infant. She is also aware that she had apparently had rubella when she was two months pregnant.

The patient did not wish to carry this pregnancy to term with the possibility of giving birth to a defective child. She asked the nurse to assist her in obtaining a legal abortion because of the high risk potential of the infant.

The nurse did not believe in abortion for any cause. She refused to assist the woman in any way to obtain the available medical service for the termination of pregnancy. The woman was able to find some assistance and to have the necessary procedure. However the nurse's refusal to assist her brought about several weeks delay and therefore made the procedure one of higher risk than if the nurse had responded to the patient's request.

a) Should the nurse's own belief be put before those of the patient's?
b) Is it ethical to withhold information of a legal available service of which the professional does not approve?
c) Do the nurse and the pre-natal service have a legal responsibility to refer the patient for the requested care?
d) Can a nurse permit herself to follow her own beliefs and not provide care for any reason whatsoever?
e) What is the nurse's professional responsibility to periodically re-examine her knowledge and beliefs which may relate to her practice, doing so in the light of scientific developments?

---

25. KNOWLEDGE OF INCORRECT TREATMENT

I am a nurse. One day a good friend and colleague came to tell me that on medical advice she had to undergo immediate surgery. She feared cancer due to the fact that in her family cases of cancer have been diagnosed too late for helpful treatment to be given. For this reason my friend used to undergo periodic examination for early diagnosis. Her fears and suspicions increased greatly when the doctor requested an interview with her husband and children before the operation.

Following the operation she showed how deep her fears were when, hardly recovered from the anaesthetic, she told me she had made her will. The abnormal size of her stomach pre-operatively and the fact that the doctor had talked with her family were to her obvious signs she had the disease she dreaded.

The result reported from the pathologist was cancer of the ovary. The eminent surgeon who had the absolute confidence of the patient, told her following the operation that he was waiting for the biopsy result for the final diagnosis as the liquid extracted from her abdomen could be caused by an illness other than cancer.

Before surgery, the doctor informed the patient's family of the probable diagnosis and that she had approximately a month to live. After the operation the diagnosis was confirmed and the estimate was further reduced to days. A different report was written out and shown to the patient, however, giving the diagnosis as tuberculosis to hide the gravity of the situation from the patient who was a nurse. Everyone close to her knew the true diagnosis but she did not.

The treatment prescribed by the surgeon was specifically for tuberculosis; medicine to be taken twice a day parenterally and medicine taken orally that a colleague and I administered to her.

The surgeon who had performed the operation then went on vacation and left another doctor in charge. Due to the holiday period this doctor was very busy and unable to visit our friend at home to perform the puncture to remove the fluid.

Up until that moment I believed I had acted in good faith. However, I began to question my conduct. I discussed the case with a specialist in gynaecological cancer and it was he who told me that if the patient followed a specific treatment for that diagnosis a better prognosis and a longer survival could be anticipated.

I decided not to participate any longer in the administration of anti-tuberculosis medication and my colleagues followed my example. I talked to the family about the consultations and they put my friend in the hands of a cancer specialist to obtain the appropriate treatment for her real diagnosis. She received the specific treatment with drugs and radiation.

She survived two years following the operation. Three months prior to her death she had to cease her normal activities. The final stage of her illness was very hard on everyone. However, we knew she received the best treatment known at the time.

Nothing was done without the knowledge of the original

surgeon. At first he was reticent to transfer the patient to the specialist, but he accepted the family's decision.

I still feel the shock of my friend's death and regret the trouble caused by my attitude.

a) Under what circumstances may a nurse intervene in the medical care of a patient?
b) What problems face a nurse who is giving professional services to a patient who is also a close personal friend?
c) Under what circumstances is it reasonable to withhold a diagnosis or other medical information from a patient?

---

26. WITHHOLDING INFORMATION TO HELP THE PATIENT

In caring for an unwed mother and her child, the public health nurse was responsible for the health of the two clients. A social worker was assigned to work with the mother in relation to her provision for the child. If the unwed mother wished to give the child up and place it for adoption the law indicated she had a certain length of time in which to make her decision. After this length of time she must retain the care and legal responsibility for the child herself.

The public health nurse learned that the social worker had made an error in telling the young mother the length of time for a decision. The public health nurse felt it would be best for the mother to make her decision in the shorter length of time. She did not correct the information for the mother, because she thought that the mother could begin adjusting to her final decision more quickly with the earlier deadline.

a) What factors should be considered by the nurse before action?
b) What is the nurse's responsibility in seeing that the social worker is informed of her mistake?
c) Should she confer with the social worker before taking any action?

d) What are the patients rights and how can they be respected?

e) What are the nurse's legal responsibilities in relation to withholding the correct information?

D. MEETING NURSING NEEDS OF PEOPLE

The code indicates that *the nurse's primary responsibility is to those people who require nursing care.* Two major issues form the basis for this statement.

First, the nurse often is in conflict caused by the needs of the patient and the interests and desires of the family, employer, or other person.

Second, who are *"people who require nursing care?"* Are they those who reach the nurse through their own efforts or by referral, or do they include persons the nurse finds and deems to be in need of care? Does the nurse, indeed, have the responsibility to find and provide care to those who lack the knowledge, will, or other resources for coming to nursing service agencies.

Some nurses may interpret the foregoing to mean that a patient's wishes regarding treatment and medication should always be honoured, and conflicts occur when health personnel do not agree on what would be best for the patient.

27. NEED FOR CONTRACEPTIVE MEASURES

A nurse was working in a family planning clinic. She spent a considerable amount of time teaching women either the necessary information regarding contraceptive techniques or that regarding optimum conditions for possible conception. She believed in planning for a small well-spaced number of children to assure the greatest potential for health of both mother and children.

More and more frequently during her work, she found she was being asked to administer a "morning-after" pill. In most instances these women did not maintain a contact with the clinic for further teaching regarding family planning. The nurse was unaware of the patients' histories and therefore questioned the seeming increase in this method of treatment. The nurse did not believe in this method of birth prevention. She did not administer this medication again.

a) What of the woman's needs could the nurse help meet?
b) What knowledge and information does the nurse need to provide more effective teaching to such women?
c) If the nurse's beliefs affect her behaviour, should she remain in the conflict situation? What can she do about it?

---

28. QUESTIONABLE PRACTICE

Miss X was hospitalized for investigation of pylonephritis. She presented a history of allergy to many drugs including several of the salicylates, the sulpha group of drugs, the penicillin group of drugs, and others.

One of the symptoms of which she complained was severe pain in the back. Routinely, Panadol and Ponstan were ordered for the relief of this pain and so they were also ordered for her. She repeated her story of the allergies to many drugs. A particular doctor "disbelieved" the patient's history of allergies to so many different drugs and believed that the patient's reactions must be psychological. He communicated this to the Sister in charge of the ward and asked to co-operate with him and offer the patient "aspirin" verbally when she administered the Panadol ordered. The Sister refused and cautioned the doctor.

During the course of events and when the Sister was not in the ward the doctor crushed two tablets of Aspirin and put them in gelatine capsules. He then called a student nurse and told her to take the capsules to Miss X. The student nurse was to explain to the patient that the capsules were new drugs for her pain and not any she had taken previously. The nurse asked the doctor the name of the drug that he had put in the capsules. She was curtly dismissed and told to carry out the order. The student nurse proceeded to take the capsules to the patient.

The patient looked suspiciously at the capsules and said the consultant who saw her that morning had not told her she was to have a new drug. She was apprehensive and made this known to the student. Instead of taking two capsules she took one and explained to the nurse that she was leery of taking new drugs because she had so many allergies and wanted to see the effect of one before taking more. The student accepted the patient's reasoning and went in search of the doctor to inform him that the patient had refused to take both capsules. She was unable to find the doctor so she went to the Sister in charge and related the whole incident to her.

Forty minutes after the patient had taken the one capsule, she called the nurse attendant and complained that she was feeling very "itchy" and was having a "tingling" feeling on her back. The Sister in charge of the ward was called. On examination, it was noticed that a fine, red, angry rash had appeared on the back below the cervical vertebrae and down as far as the sacrum in the area where she felt the "itching" and "tingling". The doctor was informed and all necessary antihistamine therapy was instituted immediately.

In the follow-up of the situation, the patient complained to the consultant that in spite of his knowledge of her allergic manifestation he had not taken sufficient precautions to prevent her from undue discomfort and possibly a dangerous reaction. Apologies were made and the patient accepted what she was told, and carried the matter no further.

The consultant reviewed the whole episode carefully and concluded the following:

The doctor had made a serious error in his

assumption that the patient's allergies were "psychological."

He had violated good medical practice by making up a gelatine capsule which was tantamount to a "misdemeanor" in this country.

He had given insufficient information to a student nurse which was a serious omission.

The student nurse was also at fault for "blindly" following orders after he refused the information.

The Sister in charge was at fault for not having reported immediately to the consultant that a junior doctor had asked her to co-operate in an "experiment" which she knew could be harmful to the patient.

He proceeded to see that the student nurse was reprimanded by the school of nursing and a record entered in her file; the Sister in Charge had a similar action taken by the Nursing Administrator; the doctor was sent a letter of warning; and the patient went home unaware of what had happened and believed that she was allergic to "just one more drug."

a) What should a student do when a doctor demands compliance to an order she questions?
b) Do the follow-up actions seem appropriate?
c) Should the patient have gone home unaware of the truth?
d) How could this incident be used by the nursing school and nursing administration to promote safer patient care?
e) What steps could be taken in the ward by the interdisciplinary team in order to ensure better care and cooperative relationships?

29. IGNORING CHILD ABUSE

A public health nurse was working with a family in the community. In caring for one member of the family, she inadvertently discovered a case of child abuse. She was well aware of the procedure to follow in a strongly suspected situation such as this. She immediately notified the physician on the local Board of Health relating all of her observations and summarizing what she felt was the problem to be treated. The physician followed the outlined procedure and the case was referred to the provincial Child Protection Agency.

The child was in Grade 7 at school. It seemed best to the case worker from the Protection Agency to go to the school to talk with this child. In the course of the interview, it became very evident that there was severe abuse of the child at home. The child, however, was very much afraid of the consequences should the case worker attempt to intervene in the home situation. The case worker decided not to pursue this problem. He carried it no further as the child had requested.

The nurse still cares for a sick member of the family. Whenever she is in the home, she sees the abuse of the child continuing.

a) What recources might the nurse use for further guidance and consultation?
b) Should she go herself to the Child Protection Agency to obtain help?
c) Should the nurse attempt to intervene with the parent who is abusing the child?
d) Are there additional persons or agencies who should be informed about the situation in the home?
e) Should the wishes of a child this age be respected as one would those of an adult?

30. REQUEST FOR NO TREATMENT

An elderly woman was readmitted to a clinic a month after her initial diagnosis and treatment for cancer had been completed. She was now obviously much worse and during the nursing admission interview mentioned several times her desire to die quickly. She expressed no interest in prolonging her life when she could not participate in familiar and enjoyable activities. Her hospitalization extended past two weeks and she did not appear to be getting any weaker. Her family persuaded her to have blood transfusions and then begin a regime of chemotherapy. She agreed. Her doctor ordered the appropriate tests, the blood transfusions, and the drugs. He also requested a surgeon to perform a venous cutdown since her veins were extremely difficult to locate for a simple venipuncture. Her doctor then went out of town for several days and transferred her to the care of another physician who had never seen her before. The chemotherapy was scheduled to begin the following morning and he proceeded as was prescribed.

The surgeon arrived and prepared to prep her leg while I was there to assist and give support. Mrs. W. started crying softly and said, "Please do not let them do this to me." The surgeon neither acknowledged her plea nor stopped working. There were also two nursing students in the room and he started explaining to them the mechanics of the cutdown procedure. I wanted to stop the entire procedure but I did not. Instead I tried to comfort Mrs. W. who proceeded to withdraw from any eye and verbal contact with me or anyone else in the room. After the cutdown was completed I stayed for a while trying to make Mrs. W. physically comfortable and allowing time for her to talk. She did not talk with me at all. When I left the room the first person I encountered was the physician temporarily in charge of her case. I vented my anger on him and he replied "What can I do?"

I spoke to the nursing students later and expressed my

feelings of frustration, helplessness, and anger at myself for not halting the cutdown in respect of her wish.

I feel I will have more courage the next time and act more on the patient's behalf; at least I hope I will.

a) Does the patient have the right to make the decision to refuse treatment?
b) How can the nurse help the patient reach a knowledgeable decision?
c) Has the nurse a responsibility to intervene on the patient's behalf in a situation like this?
d) How can the nurse utilize such a situation for teaching students and others?

CHAPTER THREE

NURSES AND PRACTICE

A. MAINTAINING STANDARDS OF PRACTICE

Most nurses have learned the basic theoretical knowledge and clinical skills in their nursing education. It is their responsibility as well as that of the employer, the association, and the educators to assure the updating of these abilities by continual education and other means. Administrative and managerial skills are frequently necessary and these abilities must be continuously improved as well as clinical knowledge and skills.

The Code recognizes that in many situations reality may impede carrying out nursing at the highest level, as stated in the set standards. Examples of such situations are: war, natural disasters, geographical isolation, inadequate or insufficient personnel, supply shortage or other material lacks, unsuitable facilities, language barrier. The following cases present conflicts of nurses in some of these situations.

---

31. PRIVATE DUTY NURSES INVOLVEMENT

Private duty nurses had been employed to care for a 95-year old gentleman who was living in a rectory, in which the priest had provided the elderly gentleman a home-like atmosphere where he could feel comfortable. The nurses had no difficulty providing him with the care he needed.

The priest had also provided quarters for a young woman who was under the care of a psychiatrist, but who was receiving additional counselling by another member of the household. This young woman had come there following surgery in a general hospital and it was known that she was addicted to hard drugs. The psychiatrist did not come to the rectory to see her, but relayed medication orders over the telephone. The orders were planned to allow gradual withdrawal from hard drugs. The nurses caring for the elderly gentleman were asked to accept these orders over the telephone and to ensure their accuracy although they had no specific responsibility for the addict nor did they give the medications to her.

The nurses were slowly drawn into the situation by virtue of one being present in the rectory at all times. The other household members kept calling upon them for help. Eventually the nurses supervised the giving of the medications and reached the point of actually giving some doses. They convinced everyone to record both the medicines administered and the young woman's behaviour.

The medication orders were changed almost daily by the doctor, and he usually asked those answering his telephone call to let him convey these orders to the nurses as they understood him more easily and could write the orders accurately. He refused to listen to the nurses' reports of the addict's behaviour when it was recorded by the non-nurse household staff.

The addict early learned to control the situation, and found ways to get increased doses of medication through the emergency orders originally intended to alleviate very severe withdrawal symptoms.

The nurses soon realized they were in a difficult position, largely of their own making. They had thought they were "helping" but suddenly they realized they were in an untenable position with no real authority to care for the "addict." Although they were concerned about the young woman, they unanimously agreed that they should no longer participate in her care in any way. The "in-house" counsellor—a priest—objected strongly to the nurses not assisting with the medication administration, and one young night nurse was unable to resist the pressure the priest placed on her to be responsible for the young woman's medications. She not only gave the medications at night, but also returned to the rectory at other times to give them. The tension this created, and the lack of sleep, soon exhausted her and she resigned from the case.

The nurses had solved their own immediate dilemma, but they had to remain in a house caring for the elderly gentleman knowing they were not giving any help to a very sick young woman—who eventually was hospitalized in a psychiatric facility and thus removed from the house.

a) To whom is the private duty nurse responsible when she becomes involved in such a "home" situation such as this one?
b) Does the private duty nurse have any responsibility, or any right, to take action related to other persons than the patient for whom she is employed, even if the other person shares the same roof or the same room?
c) How could a nurse meet such a strong "pressure" when it conflicts with her professional judgement?
d) Can an employer such as the priest in this situation add further patients to the care of nurses originally employed for one patient specifically?

---

32. MAINTAINING ASEPTIC TECHNIQUE

I am supposed to be responsible for the control and safety of techniques used in the operating theatre. I have spent many hours teaching the technicians and the aides the routines necessary for maintaining aseptic conditions during surgery. They have learned to prepare materials and to maintain an adequate supply for all needs. They have learned to handle supplies with good technique.

I find it is extremely difficult to have these appropriate routines carried out constantly by employees with little theoretical background or understanding. The surgeons are frequently breaking techniques and respond in a belligerent manner when breaks in technique are brought to their attention. I find a reminder of techniques often brings a determined response to ignore the reminder and proceed with surgery. For a male surgeon to be questioned by a female nurse is a serious breach of respect to them.

One day a surgeon wore the same gown for two successive operations even though there were other gowns available. I quietly called this to his attention, but I had no authority which really allowed me to control his behaviour for the good of the patient. In this situation even the hospital administrator was of no help to me.

a) What are the rights and responsibilities of a nurse—for other professional staff over whom she/he has no authority—for keeping to high standards of surgical asepsis?

b) What can a nurse do under such circumstances as presented in this case to insure greater safety for the patients?

---

33. ALLOCATION OF NURSING CARE TIME

On a night when the neo-natal intensive care unit was very busy and short staffed, an 800-gram premature infant was admitted. The infant had virtually no positive or stable vital signs on admission. The infant had been in the delivery suite for eight hours while the physician determined whether or not the infant could survive. Twenty minutes of concentrated effort on the part of the resident had restored a heart beat.

The heart beat was maintained for four hours and the nurse devoted much of her time caring for the infant. Her feelings in using the mechanical apparatus for suctioning, introduction of fluids, monitoring etc. were that she was mutilating the corpse of a dead infant. She also thought of the time being spent to no avail when another baby needed much care. The other infant had had corrective heart surgery and had a good prognosis for total recovery.

This nurse placed her priorities for care in prolonging life for the sickest patient rather than in assuring recovery for a patient with less urgent demands and better prognosis. She was never sure she was right.

a) Who decides priorities of time when it is limited?
b) What are the other alternatives for the nurse to consider?
c) As a basis for setting up priorities, what additional knowledge and information does the nurse need to make a decision regarding more or less care for each infant?

---

34. MAINTAINING STANDARDS OF PRACTICE

The hospital policies called for the head nurse to check all medication orders before passing them on to the medication nurse. The medication nurse normally had no direct contact with any of the physicians and did not have ready access to the full charts of patients. The medication nurse occasionally conversed with a physician if they met in or near the patient's room.

The head nurse assumed her responsibility very literally in that the medication nurse was not informed of orders until the head nurse had checked the order and passed it on to the medication nurse. The medication nurse in many instances learned that stat medication orders had been written as much as four hours before she received them. Often the reason for delay appeared to be prolonged frequent coffee breaks not just work overload. The medication nurse reported to the physician each time a stat order was unduly late, the time she had received the order and the time it was given. A full record of this was kept over a period of time and submitted to the nursing office.

This incident created considerable strain on the staff of the floor. Some felt it was inconsiderate to report a nursing superior; others felt it was basically for the good of the patients and therefore appropriate behaviour. The head nurse finally resigned her position and left the hospital. Unfortunately the hospital policy has not yet been altered to assure more efficient operation.

a) How do interpretations of hospital policies effect standards of nursing practice?
b) What is the nurse's responsibility in influencing hospital policy?
c) In this situation, were there others with whom the medication nurse should have first discussed the problem? Were there alternative steps she could have taken?

---

35. SERVICES TO THE COMMUNITY

In a small village hospital quite remote from a medical centre, elderly patients admitted to an acute medical ward following a cerebro-vascular accident and with hemiplegia are nursed over the acute stage but then they are not given rehabilitation care. The nearest establishment geared for their rehabilitation is 400 miles away and trained personnel are not available locally to implement a programme for them. However, the student nurses working in this setting are currently being instructed in depth in regard to the appropriate rehabilitation measures. They are prevented from doing any rehabilitation work with the patients in the ward by the person in charge of the unit. This has the obvious result that these people soon become completely dependent for all of their daily needs. They become placement problems for their families due to the local lack of any kind of facilities available for their care. They continue to remain in beds in the medical ward (in some instances for years) and are in a state of total dependence on the ward staff.

a) To what extent can nursing service to the community be

improved through students' services?

b) What is the instructor's role in improving service to the community?

c) What can the instructor do to encourage students to maintain high standards of care in this situation?

B. DELEGATING AND ACCEPTING RESPONSIBILITY

The nurse uses judgement in relation to individual competence when accepting and delegating responsibilities. Nurses daily face situations in which they are asked to carry out functions for which they do not feel adequately prepared, by colleagues, nursing administration, physicians, patients and families. In some instances this request may come because a more competent person is not available, in other cases it may be a question of convenience, or it might be due to lack of knowledge of the situation by the person making the request. On the other hand, the nurse may be expected to take over activities that could be done equally well by persons with less preparation, thus underutilizing nursing competencies.

In delegating activities or functions to others, the nurse must give full consideration to the dangers implicit in assignments beyond the individual's competence, as well as under-use of his potential.

36. WORK BEYOND ONE'S COMPETENCIES

I had come from the United States to a South American country to work. My Spanish was still limited although I had studied intensively for several months, in addition to my school years of reading the language.

One of the first weeks I was working at a small village hospital, a man with a gunshot wound was brought into the emergency room. It appeared that immediate surgery was necessary to try to remove the bullet and prevent infection and other complications. Several doctors conferred and I was asked to have someone prepare the patient for surgery while I scrubbed and prepared to pass instruments for the surgery.

I had never scrubbed before and did not know the names of most of the instruments in English let alone in Spanish. I refused to scrub for the surgery as there was adequate experienced staff available for this work. My refusal was considered insulting by the physician.

a) How could the nurse have reached an agreement with her colleagues (the doctors and nurses) as to the best use of her skills?
b) Should anyone else have been involved in resolving the tension between this nurse and the local doctors?
c) How did the nurse's refusal affect feelings and status of the local nursing staff?
d) Has the nurse a responsibility to inform the agency of the limits of her competency?

---

37. DELEGATING TO UNQUALIFIED HEALTH WORKERS

I was working in a country where health workers were in extremely short supply. While there were a reasonable number of doctors they congregated primarily in the large cities. Nurses with a good preparation and first level license were very scarce. The government underwrote the training of rural health aides to assist those in need of health care wherever possible in extremely deprived areas.

The young women sometimes had as little as one year of formal education before their training although most had at least three years. The course included among other things sterile techniques such as the giving of injections and changing of dressings. It also included basic treatment for endemic diseases such as malaria and tuberculosis. All of the basic routine had to be learned in six weeks and written directions were of little or no use to these students. Passing the course was made a ritual rather than an achievement. A certain number of students had to be considered graduates of the course and sent back to their home communities with full responsibilities for health care.

I was constantly living with the conflict of this quality of health care versus no health care. Was it right to delude people with the idea they were getting a trained health worker when you were sure the incorrect care was probably as common an occurrence as the correct care.

a) In a situation such as this case presents, what alternatives are available to meet the health needs?
b) Are there additional means for ensuring improved standards of care by those presently giving such care?
c) Would the nurse have been justified in refusing to participate in the situation as it is presented?
d) What are the possible outcomes of delegating independent practice to minimally qualified health workers when better prepared workers are not available?

---

38. TEACHER WORKING AS A CLERK

I am a teacher in a school of nursing. We are short of faculty and our work is further impeded because we have not found an efficient executive secretary for the school. Student records are not in order, the catalogue came out late, incorrect answers are given to enquiries. The doctor asked me to supervise the clerical staff until we found an appropriate person for the job. I agreed, even though I realized that this would infringe on my teaching and student counselling. Meanwhile, the situation has become semi-permanent. I am exhausted by trying to do two jobs and feel guilty towards the students.

a) Under what circumstances would this nurse be justified in agreeing to under-utilize her competencies?
b) What is the responsibility of the Director in relation to assignment of faculty and staff?
c) How might this situation affect other faculty, students and clerical staff?

---

39. EXPANDED NURSING ROLE

I am the only nurse in a village of 500 residents and am in charge of the Government health center. My doctor comes in for a few hours once a week. My supervisor visits me about once a month, mostly for administrative questions. I graduated a year ago and worked for six months in a similar center with an older nurse before coming here. Even though the doctor and my supervisor can be reached by phone, when I asked them for advice, I am not sure that my analysis of the patient's condition is complete or correct. I was not taught to do physical examinations and legally I am not allowed to prescribe medicines. Yet they tell me to do my best. One day I will make a serious mistake. The tension is great and yet it is a challenge to fill this role.

a) In what ways could this nurse obtain help?
b) What is the responsibility of the government to the villagers?
c) What is the responsibility of the nurse in relation to her "expanded role?"

CHAPTER FOUR

NURSES AND CO-WORKERS

A. COOPERATIVE RELATIONSHIPS

Under the heading, *Nurses and Co-Workers,* the Code for Nurses states *the nurse sustains a cooperative relationship with co-workers in nursing and other fields.* The relationship between nurses and other workers; however, often leaves much to be desired. Within nursing itself, the traditional hierarchy often is interpreted as "there are those who give the orders, and those who carry out orders." In a truly cooperative relationship, especially between staff and administration, there should be "give and take" all around. Between nurses and doctors, the relationship is often one of clear subordination and domination, with nurses frequently tending to find unobtrusive ways of working with patients actively but without impinging on the doctor's "superior" role. This may be interpreted as a "harmonious relationship," but truly professional nursing calls for a true colleague relationship with information sharing as well as decision making with nurses, doctors, and other workers involved in some aspect of patient care and well being.

---

40. REPORTING A STUDENT NURSE ILLNESS

One afternoon at around 2:15 p.m. a relief ward sister walked to a ward and found the only nurse available on duty in the sluice room, crying. She was a student enrolled nurse. The ward sister asked her to explain why she was behaving in that manner. The young nurse related how she had gone to report to the Matron that she was not well and did not feel able to work that afternoon. The Matron had sent her back to work as she was the only nurse available to care for that unit. She also told the student that sick nurses are supposed to report their sickness first thing in the morning and not in the afternoon.

Having heard the nurse's story the ward sister decided to check her pulse and temperature and found that both were much raised. As a result of these findings the ward sister decided to take the nurse to the doctor. When he examined her, he diagnosed her as suffering from acute tonsillitis and malaria. The nurse was admitted right away and put on treatment for these conditions.

The ward sister then reported to the Matron that the student nurse she had sent back on duty had been admitted with the above diagnosis. The Matron was very displeased that the ward sister had acted on her own. From that day on, the Matron developed a very hostile relationship with the ward sister concerned. The ward sister does not know how to improve their relationship so they can work well together.

a) What alternatives did the ward sister have in dealing with the student's problem?
b) In such a situation, what is the ward sister's major responsibility?
c) How can good relationships be re-established?
d) What implications are there in sending a sick student nurse to the ward?
e) How might this incident influence the future relationships of the students?

---

41. LACK OF APPROPRIATE NURSING HISTORY

Last year I was working on a project in which I was studying the effectiveness of the teaching of diabetic patients. I came across the following situation.

A 32-year old woman worker came to the clinic for her yearly physical examination. The doctor tentatively made a diagnosis of diabetes which was soon confirmed after the appropriate tests. She was admitted to the hospital for the period of regulation of her diet and insulin. When her condition was stabilized, she was taught the mechanics of providing herself with the correct diet and dosage of insulin. She appeared to grasp the new knowledge quickly and was discharged.

She returned to her home and work and I visited her at home to evaluate the effectiveness of the teaching. She was not progressing as well as we had expected and I reviewed all of the care with her. Much to my surprise I found that her insulin was calculated correctly and her diet also. The problem I identified was: she was working, and therefore eating at night but taking her insulin at 7 a.m. before she went to sleep.

I proceeded with my teaching to help her adjust to the appropriate regimen for her. While I said nothing to reflect upon my professional colleagues directly I could hardly give the proper care without it reflecting adversely upon my colleagues in the mind of this patient.

a) What alternative steps could the nurse have taken when identifying the patient's problem?
b) What is a nurse/researcher's responsibility in relation to the population being studied?
c) Could the care be given without reflecting adversely on the professional colleagues?
d) Should the researcher try to influence the practices in the institution?

---

42. ASSESSMENT OF A CHILD'S HEARING

Because of problems a child was having in school, the public health nurse requested a clinic physician to assess the child's hearing. This clinic physician then referred the child on to a specialized institution for further assessment.

He also forwarded all the information to the child's private paediatrician recommending a neurological assessment.

When the nurse checked with the child's teacher about his progress she learned that the mother had been told by the paediatrician that the public health nurse should "mind her own business" and not try to usurp the paediatrician's role. The paediatrician also stated that the child should continue in the regular school system. However, the special hearing Institute found a marked bilateral hearing loss requiring two hearing aids. They recommended that the child should attend a special education programme for at least a period of time until his problems were resolved. The nurse was placed in conflict as to how to proceed with the follow-up for this child.

a) What advice, if any, should she give the parents?
b) What should she say to the child's private paediatrician to resolve the conflict?
c) What course of action might the nurse have taken to prevent this conflict?

B. SAFEGUARDING THE PATIENT

The nurse takes appropriate action to safeguard the individual when his care is endangered by a co-worker or any other person. The nurse will recall vividly those times when it appears that the patient is in danger due to some one else's actions. The nurse also may find the conflict particularly difficult when the other health worker is a physician. Extenuating circumstances often pressure the nurse to take certain actions which may not be deemed to be best for the patient. Examples of conflicts of personnel and the traumatic effect on the nurse is illustrated in these reports.

43. FREE USE OF RESTRAINTS

Working in a psychiatric emergency room a nurse witnessed a very angry and aggressive young woman being literally dragged in by her father and brother. The patient appeared to be irrational. She was definitely resisting and fighting in a violent and vehement manner the attempt of her family to bring her in to the hospital. Finally after the scene continued for about 15 minutes, the doctor ordered the nurse to restrain all four limbs of the patient and to sedate her. The orderlies dragged the patient into an emergency room alcove where there was a stretcher which had four restraints attached to it. The orderlies had to hold her down with very strong armed tactics. The nurse proceeded to carry out the doctor's order, although she was apparently doing this very reluctantly.

What disturbed the nurse the most was the fact that, to her knowledge, no one even attempted to communicate or listen to the patient. The nurse had not been given any opportunity to do so and no one else seemed to try. She was quite sure the need for the restraints was not documented well enough.

a) Whose needs were being met? the patient's? the family's? or the staff's?
b) What is the nurse's responsibility in such a situation?
c) In addition to carrying out "the doctor's orders," was there something more she could have done?
d) Under what circumstances might the nurse approve of the use of restraints?

44. CENSORING MAIL OF THE PSYCHIATRIC PATIENT

While working on a psychiatric unit I was expected to review the mail of all my assigned patients and also when possible to monitor their phone calls. In doing this I frequently knew that the patient was expressing thoughts in these communications that he/she was not revealing in therapeutic sessions. These thoughts were then duly recorded in the patient's record for the information of those concerned with the patient's treatment. There were probably numerous times when these pieces of information may have helped the therapist understand the patient and therefore do better work. It certainly appeared to be a contributing factor toward better care for the patient.

As I proceeded to do this, I wondered about the ethics involved. I was concerned whether or not a patient's illness gives us adequate reason to deprive him of his rights and privacy one usually accords a human being. Even when these communications may contain threats to individuals or plans for inappropriate actions of some kind I was not sure if we were justified in censoring mail and phone calls.

a) Under the guise of "the welfare of the patient" are we going beyond our rights as therapist for disturbed patients?
b) Where is the line between information seeking for patient care planning and intrusion of privacy, particularly with the psychiatric patient?
c) What procedural guidelines can help safeguard the patient's privacy?
d) Is censoring patient's mail and telephone calls materially different from observing the patient or encouraging him to express himself?

---

45. PHYSICIAN'S NON-RESPONSE TO A CALL FROM A NURSE

As a new staff nurse, I was caring for a seriously ill patient who had a cardiac monitor attached. I was the only first level nurse on the unit when I noticed a change in the wave pattern on the monitor. My expertise was not adequate to categorize the specific change and there was no one there on the unit to help me. I called the supervisor who said she was too busy to come to the unit but that I should call the resident physician. I asked the telephone operator to page him and I returned to the patient.

There was no apparent change in the vital signs but the patient's restlessness became quite obvious and concerned me greatly. Although the resident had not answered his page, I finally located him in the emergency room. All I could tell him was the wave was different and I thought he should come and check the patient as I was not experienced enough to interpret the change. In about thirty minutes, the vital signs began to change drastically and I placed an emergency call to the resident to come immediately. He still had not arrived when I had to place a general emergency call because of the need for cardiac resuscitation. By the time he arrived his only duty was to pronounce the death of the patient.

I was off for the next two nights and when I returned I talked with the supervisor about reporting the lack of response from the resident. I felt that an investigation would establish whether he was negligent in his care or if the staffing was inadequate to cope with emergencies. She told me to forget the incident, an investigation would cause me a lot of unnecessary discomfort and be time consuming. Without her support I did not press the issue.

I later learned that the patient died of a massive haemorrhage of an abdominal aneurism and probably nothing could have been done to prevent his death.

I knew that the patient could not have been saved, but I resigned from the institution very disillusioned.

a) What actions should be taken to prevent similar incidents in the future?
b) What are the ethical issues in this case?
c) Did the nurse's resignation solve any of the problems?
d) Does the irreversible condition of the patient alter the responsibility of any party?

46. A CRITICALLY INJURED PATIENT

I was working in a community hospital with a limited number of medical specialists on the staff. We relied upon consultants from a nearby medical centre for some specialties. A patient was admitted to the emergency room one night with an obvious depressed skull fracture caused by assault with apparent intent to murder. The supervisor saw the immediate need for a neurosurgeon. She had great difficulty in reaching one, the time being Saturday night shortly after midnight.

Three neurosurgeons were contacted by telephone. The first two stated that they were not on call that night and rang off. The third wanted the patient who at this time was virtually moribund, to be transferred to the medical centre closer to the physician's home. He would see him there. The supervisor refused to allow the patient to be transferred because of his critical condition, and so told the physician. He still would not respond to her request by coming to see the patient. However, half an hour later he called the supervisor back. This time he requested that the patient be transferred to a medical centre where he could be held so that his kidneys could be removed for transplant at the time of his death. She again refused to honour this request and continued to seek a neurosurgeon who would come to evaluate the patient's condition.

This nurse questioned her own judgement after the patient expired. I feel she acted in the best interest of the patient. She wondered if she should have risked the transfer of the patient as the only possible hope for him, since no physician could be found who would come to the patient.

a) Should a nurse cooperate with the physician to help provide a source of organs for transplant?
b) What could have been this nurse's considerations in questioning her own judgement?
c) On making such a decision, what additional steps could

the supervision of the emergency room have taken?
d) What steps can be taken to prevent a repetition of such incidents?

---

47. PROBLEMS OF AN OBSTETRICAL PATIENT

Mrs. B. was a patient with a history of difficult obstetrical problems. She had been married for 10 years and had had 4 abortions in that time. She had never born a viable child and it was discovered she had an incompetent cervix. A Shirodikor Stitch was inserted at 16 weeks of her current pregnancy and it was supposed to be removed at 36 weeks or at least at the onset of labour.

Mrs. B. was admitted into the labour ward at 36 weeks with labour pains which had started 2-3 hours before her arrival at the hospital. The midwife informed the doctor on duty, who came and saw the patient and confirmed labour. The Shirodikor Stitch still in the midwife reminded the doctor that it should be removed but no action was taken. The instructions given by the doctor were for the nurse to "observe the patient."

The patient laboured on and the cervical os became fully dilated in the next 2 hours. At that time, the midwife reviewed the patient and she observed vaginal bleeding and that the patient was bearing down. The doctor was again called urgently but by the time he saw the patient she had pushed the baby out and was in a state of shock. She had lost a lot of blood. The baby appeared asphyxiated; it was incubated but eventually died apparently as a result of oxygen deprivation.

The mother was taken to the operating theatre for exploration of the uterus which was found torn longitudinally from the cervix to the fundus. Immediately a hysterectomy was done. After all that had occurred, the doctor wrote in the patient's chart that no scissors were presented to him, and therefore he could not remove the Shirodikor Stitch. The midwife and her colleagues related their actions carefully in the chart and to the chief of medicine. They did not feel the doctor's charted comments were appropriate nor that he should have implied they were responsible for the problems.

a) What should a nurse do when she feels she is unjustly accused?
b) What additional steps could the nurse have taken to safeguard the patient at the time of delivery?
c) What are the legal implications and are the nurses involved?

---

48. QUESTIONING THE DOCTOR'S ORDERS

I was caring for a patient who was in serious distress from an asthma condition. It was obvious he needed medical attention. I called his doctor and she gave no medical orders over the phone but instead came immediately to the hospital. When the doctor arrived she was obviously intoxicated. She left several orders for the patient. Some of the orders appeared to me and the other nurses as appropriate and some were definitely inappropriate and would possibly be harmful to the patient if given as ordered.

The patient's care was uppermost in my mind, but I also knew that the legal responsibility to order specific medications was the doctor's. In this case the patient's doctor was obviously in no condition to review the orders with me and hear my opinion as to the reasons they were inappropriate. For the patient's safety, my knowledge of pharmacology made me certain I should not given them. The other nurses on the unit agreed with me.

I consulted with other doctors who were present and knew of the dilemma. They had observed the condition of the doctor and also agreed that the orders were inappropriate. They refused, however, to take or even suggest any steps to resolve the problem.

Finally the nurses definitely decided we should refuse to

follow the doctor's orders. The nurses took turns staying constantly with the patient. We used whatever nursing measures we could to ease his condition. The other nurses spent a long time telephoning until finally the chief of the medical staff was contacted. When he arrived he made certain the appropriate medical care was ordered. The patient soon had relief.

a) Is it the nurses responsibility to see that policies are written to guide them in this situation?
b) Was there an alternative course of action for the nurses?

---

49. REPORT OF AN ACCIDENT

Five or six years ago I was working for a modern Southern European passenger line. As we approached her port of disembarkation, a passenger came into the hospital with an obvious Colle's fracture. I made out the accident form while waiting for the surgeon to come. He ordered an Xray. To my surprise he said the Xray showed no sign of a fracture. The patient went ashore with her arm in a sling.

Nobody thought anything more about the case until the next time the ship reached the same port. Then an agent reported that, not satisfied with the care that had been given for her arm, the patient had ultimately gone to another doctor. This doctor had diagnosed a Colle's fracture and proceeded to treat her for this. She was going to sue the shipping line. The form I had written was unearthed and I was told to write it and omit my remark "Colle's fracture."

a) What are the ethical implications, both personal and professional, of changing a report?
b) What are the legal implications of agreeing to change the report?
c) What steps might the nurse take in regard to the company, the patient, and herself?

50. ALLERGIC REACTION TO A TRANSFUSION

Mr. Y. was a patient who was admitted to the hospital with a diagnosis of severe iron-deficiency anaemia (Haemoglobin 4 gms). The treatment sheet showed that 2 pints of blood were to be given to the patient first. If there were no symptoms of reaction a further 2 pints were to be administered after a haemoglobin estimation was made.

Mr. Y. was in one of four side rooms of a 22-bed male medical ward. His general condition seemed poor. He looked quite emaciated, weak and very ill. His weight was recorded as 120 lbs., height 5′9″ and blood pressure 80/60.

The staff of the ward at the time included a second year student, one first year student, and one registered nurse who had to service an equally large female medical ward in addition to the male ward.

A junior doctor came to the ward and started the transfusion. The second year student who was assisting the doctor, started a quarter hourly observation chart. After two hours, during which time there was a gradual but slow increase in the pulse and the blood pressure, the patient complained of feeling "unwell." The student nurse slowed the drip (from 30 drops a minute to about 10 drops) and went to look for the registered nurse. The patient was reassessed by the registered nurse and the transfusion reset at 30 drops per minute.

The first pint of the blood transfusion was completed in five hours. The junior doctor visited the patient and was informed by a staff nurse that the patient was showing signs of a reaction as supported by the observation chart recordings. He ordered the second pint be commenced remarking "the reaction is too mild to be of concern."

By the time the second pint of blood was completed, the patient's temperature was elevated by 1°C and the patient continued to feel "unwell." The junior doctor was again informed and the nurse suggested no further blood be given.

This time he remarked that the nurses should stop challenging the doctors and they should just carry out orders. He told them to add the third pint and continue later with the fourth. The nurses did give the third pint of blood and also the fourth. By this time the patient was having rigours, hyperpyrexia, pain in the loins and sweating. Subsequently he collapsed. It was necessary to have the patient transferred to a special care unit immediately where it took him 72 hours to recover from the ill effects of the transfusion.

Unfortunately, the nurses never learned what the follow-up of this situation was.

a) What could the nurse have done to maintain her professional judgement and safeguard the patient's health?
b) In retrospect, what could the nurse do to prevent a repetition of such a situation?
c) Should the nurse be concerned about safeguarding herself legally. If so, what steps would she take to do so?

CHAPTER FIVE

NURSES AND THE PROFESSION

A. SOCIAL AND ECONOMIC WORKING CONDITIONS

In the past decade ICN has promoted improved salary and work conditions for nurses. The Council has helped member associations develop programs to achieve conditions for nurses in their countries which are equitable to those of persons who have similar qualifications and responsibilities. On the international level, ICN worked with the World Health Organization and the International Labour Organization to prepare a document* which hopefully will have a major impact on recruiting and retaining nurses in the work force.

The change in the status of the nurse in modern times from a single woman living in a nurses' residence, to a married male or female nurse, required changes in conditions of employment.

The Code states that *the nurse, acting through the professional organization, participates in establishing and maintaining equitable social and economic working conditions in nursing.*

---

*ILO-WHO "Joint meeting on Conditions of Work and Life of Nursing Personnel, Geneva, Nov. 19-30, 1973." ILO Report VI (II) "Employment and Conditions of Work and life of Nursing Personnel", Geneva, 1977.

51. A NURSING STRIKE

I am a supervisor in a general hospital near my home. The nurses in another hospital in this city are on strike. There are many issues of controversy but a major one is the denial of the nurses' request to have a voice in policy-making which has a direct effect on nursing care. The nurses association is the unit the nurses wish to represent them as their bargaining agent but the hospital will not recognize them as such.

Like several association officers, I am showing my support by encouraging the striking group at times when I am not on duty in my own position. I was also interviewed by the press and quoted as being in support of the striking nurses. My employer has requested that I stop all supportive activities because the public may interpret my action as a criticism of my own employing hospital. We do have a voice in policy-making where I am employed and I think it helps us improve the care to patients. I wish to help my colleagues obtain the same privileges in their place of employment.

a) How can this nurse explain her concept of her professional responsibility as an association member?
b) Are there ways the association can help this nurse's relationship with her own employer?
c) What are the implications for her employing institution if the public interprets her action as the employer suggests they might?

52. A NEW IMMIGRANT NURSE

I am an immigrant nurse living but one year in this country. I have not been able to get a work permit as a registered nurse because I did not pass the examinations of this new country although I sat for them twice. My family is in a difficult financial situation, and I must send money to them.

The owner of a small private hospital, whom I met socially, asked me to work in his hospital under the title of nurse aide on condition that I carry the responsibility of the senior nurse on night duty. I know that I could do this work competently and safely as I had a good training and many years of experience in similar hospital nursing. However, it is clear that I am being cheated of the proper salary, and also asked to break the law by doing work of a nurse while carrying another title. In addition, accepting these conditions will contribute to the exploitation of nurses. I have decided to take the job, but am very uncomfortable about it.

a) Who should have helped this nurse?
b) Should she have found other ways to meet her financial needs?
c) Was there any additional action she could have taken?

---

53. MEMBERSHIP IN A PROFESSIONAL ASSOCIATION

I am a Registered Nurse with a master's degree, working in a senior nursing position in the Ministry of Health. Compared to other professionals at the same level, my salary and working conditions are much lower. It has been suggested that I join the association of academic administrative workers which would greatly improve my conditions—but if I did so I would have to leave the Nurses' Association. My decision to leave the Association might influence other nurses with academic degrees to follow in my steps. I am in a conflict—should my personal needs override my allegiance to the Nurses' Association.

a) What other alternatives are there for this nurse?
b) Whose responsibility is it to try to solve this problem?
c) Is this nurse's status affected by receiving a lower salary than her non-nursing colleagues?

READING A

FLORENCE NIGHTINGALE PLEDGE FOR NURSES

I solemnly pledge myself before God and in the presence of this assembly to pass my life in purity and to practise my profession faithfully.

I will abstain from whatever is deleterious and mischievous, and will not take or knowingly administer any harmful drug.

I will do all in my power to elevate the standard of my profession, and will hold in confidence all personal matters committed to my keeping, and all family affairs coming to my knowledge in the practice of my calling.

With loyalty will I endeavour to aid the physician in his work, and devote myself to the welfare of those committed to my care.

> *"The Florence Nightingale Pledge was prepared by a special committee appointed by the Farrand Training School Committee of Harper Hospital, Detroit, in 1893 . . . The name was selected because it represents the highest type of nurse and an ideal."*

quote from: Editorial comment: American Journal of Nursing 11(10): 777, July 11, USA.

READING B

INTERNATIONAL CODE OF NURSING ETHICS 1953

Professional nurses minister to the sick, assume responsibility for creating a physical, social and spiritual environment which will be conducive to recovery, and stress the prevention of illness and promotion of health by teaching and example. They render health-service to the individual, the family, and the community and co-ordinate their services with members of other health professions.

Service to mankind is the primary function of nurses and the reason for the existence of the nursing profession. Need for nursing service is universal. Professional nursing service is therefore unrestricted by consideration of nationality, race, creed, colour, politics or social status.

Inherent in the code is the fundamental concept that the nurse believes in the essential freedoms of mankind and in the preservation of human life.

The profession recognises that an international code cannot cover in detail all the activities and relationships of nurses, some of which are conditioned by personal philosophies and beliefs.

1. The fundamental responsibility of the nurse is threefold: to conserve life, to alleviate suffering and to promote health.
2. The nurse must maintain at all times the highest standards of nursing care and of professional conduct.
3. The nurse must not only be well prepared to practise, but must maintain her knowledge and skill at a consistently high level.
4. The religious beliefs of a patient must be respected.
5. Nurses hold in confidence all personal information entrusted to them.

Adopted by the Grand Council of the International Council of Nurses, Sao Paulo, Brazil, July 10, 1953.

6. A nurse recognises not only the responsibilities but the limitations of her or his professional functions; recommends or gives medical treatment without medical orders only in emergencies and reports such action to a physician at the earliest possible moment.
7. The nurse is under an obligation to carry out the physician's orders intelligently and loyally and to refuse to participate in unethical procedures.
8. The nurse sustains confidence in the physician and other members of the health team; incompetence or unethical conduct of associates should be exposed but only to the proper authority.
9. A nurse is entitled to just remuneration and accepts only such compensation as the contract, actual or implied, provides.
10. Nurses do not permit their names to be used in connection with the advertisement of products or with any other forms of self-advertisement.
11. The nurse co-operates with and maintains harmonious, relationships with members of other professions and with her or his nursing colleagues.
12. The nurse in private life adheres to standards of personal ethics which reflect credit upon the profession.
13. In personal conduct nurses should not knowingly disregard the accepted patterns of behaviour of the community in which they live and work.
14. A nurse should participate and share responsibility with other citizens and other health professions in promoting efforts to meet the health needs of the public—local, state, national and international.

READING C

ROLE OF THE NURSE IN THE CARE OF DETAINEES AND PRISONERS

WHEREAS the ICN *Code for Nurses* specifically states that

1. "The fundamental responsibility of the nurse is fourfold: to promote health, to prevent illness, to restore health and to alleviate suffering.
2. "The nurse's primary responsibility is to those people who require nursing care.
3. "The nurse when acting in a professional capacity should at all times maintain standards of personal conduct which reflect credit upon the profession.
4. "The nurse takes appropriate action to safeguard the individual when his care is endangered by a co-worker or any other person," and

WHEREAS in 1973 ICN reaffirmed support for the Red Cross Rights and Duties of Nurses under the Geneva Conventions of 1949, which specifically state that, in case of armed conflict of international as well as national character (i.e. internal disorders, civil wars, armed rebellions):

1. Members of the armed forces, prisoners and persons taking no active part in the hostilities
   a) shall be entitled to protection and care if wounded or sick,
   b) shall be treated humanely, that is:
   — they may not be subjected to physical mutilation or to medical or scientific experiments of any kind which are not justified by the medical, dental or hospital treatment of the prisoner concerned and carried out in his interest,
   — they shall not be wilfully left without medical assistance and care, nor shall conditions exposing them to contagion or infection be created,
   — they shall be treated humanely and cared for by the Party in conflict in whose power they may be, without adverse distinction founded on sex, race, nationality, religion, political opinion, or any other similar criteria.

Policy Statement adopted by the Council of Representatives of the International Council of Nurses, Singapore, August 1975.

2. The following acts are and shall remain prohibited at any time and in any place whatsoever with respect to the above-mentioned persons:
   a) violence to life and person, in particular murder of all kinds, mutilation, cruel treatment and torture;
   b) outrages upon personal dignity, in particular humiliating and degrading treatment.

WHEREAS in 1971 ICN endorsed the United Nations Universal Declaration of Human Rights and, hence, accepted that

1. "Everyone is entitled to all the rights and freedoms, set forth in this Declaration, without distinction of any kind, such as race, colour, sex, language, religion, political or other opinion, national or social origin, property, birth or other status (Art. 2),
2. "No one shall be subjected to torture or to cruel, inhuman or degrading treatment or punishment (Art. 5);" and

WHEREAS in relation to detainees and prisoners of conscience, interrogation procedures are increasingly being employed which result in ill effects, often permanent, on the person's mental and physical health;

THEREFORE BE IT RESOLVED that ICN condemns the use of all such procedures harmful to the mental and physical health of prisoners and detainees; and

FURTHER BE IT RESOLVED that nurses having knowledge of physical or mental ill-treatment of detainees and prisoners take appropriate action including reporting the matter to appropriate national and/or international bodies; and

FURTHER BE IT RESOLVED that nurses participate in clinical research carried out on prisoners, only if the freely given consent of the patient has been secured after a complete explanation and understanding by the patient of the nature and risk of the research; and

FINALLY BE IT RESOLVED that the nurse's first responsibility is towards her patients, notwithstanding considerations of national security and interest.

READING D

CODE FOR NURSES WITH INTERPRETATIVE STATEMENTS

INTRODUCTION

The development of a code of ethics is an essential characteristic of a profession and provides one means for the exercise of professional self-regulation. A code indicates a profession's acceptance of the responsibility and trust with which it has been invested by society. Upon entering the profession of nursing, each person inherits a measure of the responsibility and trust that has accrued to nursing over the years and the corresponding obligation to adhere to the profession's code of conduct and relationships for ethical practice.

The *Code for Nurses,* adopted by the American Nurses' Association in 1950 and periodically revised, serves to inform both the nurse and society of the profession's expectations and requirements in ethical matters. The *Code* and the Interpretive Statements together provide a framework for the nurse to make ethical decisions and discharge responsibilities to the public, to other members of the health team, and to the profession. While it is impossible to anticipate in a code every type of situation that may be encountered in professional practice, the direction and suggestions provided here are widely applicable.

The *Code for Nurses* and the Interpretive Statements are both directed toward present-day practice. Previous *Codes* have been more prescriptive, identifying codes of both personal and professional behavior, describing appropriate relationships with physicians and other health professionals, and identifying certain responsibilities of the nurse as a citizen, an employee, and a person. The present *Code,* while remaining prescriptive, depends more on the nurse's accountability to the client, and, in that sense, represents a change to an ethical code.

The requirements of the *Code* may often exceed, but are never less than those of the law. While violations of the law may subject the nurse to civil or criminal liability, the constituent associations may reprimand, censure, suspend, or expel ANA members from the Association for violations of the *Code.* The possible loss of the respect and confidence of society and one's colleagues are serious sanctions which may result from violation of

---

the *Code*. Each nurse has a personal obligation to uphold and adhere to the *Code* and to insure that nursing colleagues do likewise. Guidance and assistance in implementing the *Code* in local situations may be obtained from the American Nurses' Association or its state constituents.

PREAMBLE

The *Code for Nurses* is based on belief about the nature of individuals, nursing, health, and society. Recipients and providers of nursing services are viewed as individuals and groups who possess basic rights and responsibilities, and whose values and circumstances command respect at all times. Nursing encompasses the promotion and restoration of health, the prevention of illness, and the alleviation of suffering. The statements of the *Code* and their interpretation provide guidance for conduct and relationships in carrying out nursing responsibilities consistent with the ethical obligations of the profession and quality in nursing care.

CODE FOR NURSES

1 The nurse provides services with respect for human dignity and the uniqueness of the client unrestricted by considerations of social or economic status, personal attributes, or the nature of health problems.

2 The nurse safeguards the client's right to privacy by judiciously protecting information of a confidential nature.

3 The nurse acts to safeguard the client and the public when health care and safety are affected by the incompetent, unethical, or illegal practice of any person.

4 The nurse assumes responsibility and accountability for individual nursing judgments and actions.

5 The nurse maintains competence in nursing.

6 The nurse exercises informed judgment and uses individual competence and qualifications as criteria in seeking consultation, accepting responsibilities, and delegating nursing activities to others.

7 The nurse participates in activities that contribute to the ongoing development of the profession's body of knowledge.

8 The nurse participates in the profession's efforts to implement and improve standards of nursing.

9 The nurse participates in the profession's efforts to establish and maintain conditions of employment conducive to high quality nursing care.

10 The nurse participates in the profession's effort to protect the public from misinformation and misrepresentation and to maintain the integrity of nursing.

11 The nurse collaborates with members of the health professions and other citizens in promoting community and national efforts to meet the health needs of the public.

CODE FOR NURSES WITH INTERPRETIVE STATEMENTS

1. THE NURSE PROVIDES SERVICES WITH RESPECT FOR HUMAN DIGNITY AND THE UNIQUENESS OF THE CLIENT UNRESTRICTED BY CONSIDERATIONS OF SOCIAL OR ECONOMIC STATUS, PERSONAL ATTRIBUTES, OR THE NATURE OF HEALTH PROBLEMS.

1.1 SELF-DETERMINATION OF CLIENTS

Whenever possible, clients should be fully involved in the planning and implementation of their own health care. Each client has the moral right to determine what will be done with his/her person; to be given the information necessary for making informed judgments; to be told the possible effects of care; and to accept, refuse, or terminate treatment. These same rights apply to minors and others not legally qualified and must be respected to the fullest degree permissible under the law. The law in these areas may differ from state to state; each nurse has an obligation to be knowledgeable about and to protect and support the moral and legal rights of all clients under state laws and applicable federal laws, such as the 1974 Privacy act.

The nurse must also recognize those situations in which individual rights to self-determination in health care may temporarily be altered for the common good. The many variables involved make it imperative that each case be considered with full awareness of the need to provide for informed judgments while preserving the rights of clients.

1.2 SOCIAL AND ECONOMIC STATUS OF CLIENTS

The need for nursing care is universal, cutting across all national, ethnic, religious, cultural, political, and economic differences, as does nursing's responses to this fundamental need. Nursing care should be determined solely by human need, irrespective of background, circumstances, or other indices of individual social and economic status.

1.3 PERSONAL ATTRIBUTES OF CLIENTS

Age, sex, race, color, personality, or other personal attributes, as well as individual differences in background, customs, attitudes, and beliefs, influence nursing practice only insofar as they represent factors the nurse must understand, consider, and respect in tailoring care to personal needs and in maintaining the individual's self-respect and dignity. Consideration of individual value systems and lifestyles should be included in the planning of health care for each client.

1.4 THE NATURE OF HEALTH PROBLEMS

The nurse's respect for the worth and dignity of the individual human being applies irrespective of the nature of the health problem. It is reflected in the care given the person who is disabled as well as the normal; the patient with the long-term illness as well as the one with the acute illness, or the recovering patient as well as the one who is terminally ill or dying. It extends to all who require the services of the nurse for the promotion of health, the prevention of illness, the restoration of health, and the alleviation of suffering.

The nurse's concern for human dignity and the provision of quality nursing care is not limited by personal attitudes or beliefs. If personally opposed to the delivery of care in a particular case because of the nature of the health problem or the procedures to be used, the nurse is justified in refusing to participate. Such refusal should be made known in advance and in time for other appropriate arrangements to be made for the client's nursing care. If the nurse must knowingly enter such a case under emergency circumstances or enters unknowingly, the obligation to provide the best possible care is observed. The nurse withdraws from this type of situation only when assured that alternative sources of nursing care are available to the client. If a client requests information or counsel in an area that is legally sanctioned but contrary to the nurse's personal beliefs, the nurse may refuse to provide these services but must advise the client of sources where such service is available.

1.5 THE SETTING FOR HEALTH CARE

The nurse adheres to the principle of non-discriminatory, non-prejudicial care in every employment setting or situation and endeavors to promote its acceptance by others. The nurse's readiness to accord respect to clients and to render or obtain needed services should not be limited by the setting, whether nursing care is given in an acute care hospital, nursing home, drug or alcoholic treatment center, prison, patient's home, or other setting.

1.6 THE DYING PERSON

As the concept of death and ways of dealing with it changes, the basic human values remain. The ethical problems posed, however, and the decision-making responsibilities of the patient, family, and professional are increased.

The nurse seeks ways to protect these values while working with the client and others to arrive at the best decisions dictated by the circumstances, the client's rights and wishes, and the highest standards of care. The measures used to provide assistance should enable the client to live with as much comfort, dignity, and freedom from anxiety and pain as possible. The client's nursing care will determine to a great degree how this final human experience is lived and the peace and dignity with which death is approached.

2. THE NURSE SAFEGUARDS THE CLIENT'S RIGHT TO PRIVACY BY JUDICIOUSLY PROTECTING INFORMATION OF A CONFIDENTIAL NATURE.

2.1 DISCLOSURE TO THE HEALTH TEAM

It is an accepted standard of nursing practice that data about the health status of clients be accessible, communicated, and recorded. Provision of quality health services requires that such data be available to all members of the health team. When knowledge gained in confidence is relevant or essential to others involved in planning or implementing the client's care, professional judgment is used in sharing it. Only information pertinent to a client's treatment and welfare is disclosed and only to those directly concerned with the client's care. The rights, well-being, and safety of the individual client should be the determining factors in arriving at this decision.

2.2 DISCLOSURE FOR QUALITY ASSURANCE PURPOSES

Patient information required to document the appropriateness, necessity, and quality of care that is required for peer review, third party payment, and other quality assurance mechanisms must be disclosed only under rigidly defined policies, mandates, or protocols. These written guidelines must assure that the confidentiality of client information is maintained.

2.3 DISCLOSURE TO OTHERS NOT INVOLVED IN THE CLIENT'S CARE

The right of privacy is an inalienable right of all persons, and the nurse has a clear obligation to safeguard any confidential information about the client acquired from any source. The nurse-client relationship is built on trust. This relationship could be destroyed and the clients' welfare and reputation jeopardized by injudicious disclosure of information provided in confidence. Since the concept of confidentiality has legal as well as ethical implications, an inappropriate breach of confidentiality may also expose the nurse to liability.

2.4 DISCLOSURE IN A COURT OF LAW

Occasionally, the nurse may be obligated to give testimony in a court of law in relation to confidential information about a client. This should be done only under proper authorization or legal compulsion. Privilege in relation to the disclosure of such information is a legal right that only the patient or his representative may claim or waive. The statutes governing privilege and the exceptions to them vary from state to state, and the nurse may wish to consult legal counsel before testifying in court to be fully informed about professional rights and responsibilities.

2.5 ACCESS TO RECORDS

If, in the course of providing care, there is need for access to the records of persons not under the nurse's care, as may be the case in relation to the records of the mother of a newborn, the person should be notified and permission first obtained whenever possible. Although records belong to the agency where collected, the individual maintains the right of control over the information provided by him, his family, and his environment. Similarly, professionals may exercise the right of control over information generated by them in the course of health care.

If the nurse wishes to use a client's treatment record for research or nonclinical purposes in which confidential information may be identified, the client's consent must first be obtained. Ethically, this insures the client's right to privacy; legally, it serves to protect the client against unlawful invasion of privacy and the nurse against liability for such action.

3. THE NURSE ACTS TO SAFEGUARD THE CLIENT AND THE PUBLIC WHEN HEALTH CARE AND SAFETY ARE AFFECTED BY INCOMPETENT, UNETHICAL, OR ILLEGAL PRACTICE OF ANY PERSON.

3.1 ROLE OF ADVOCATE

The nurse's primary commitment is to the client's care and safety. Hence, in the role of client advocate, the nurse must be alert to and take appropriate action regarding any instances of incompetent, unethical, or illegal practice(s) by any member of the health care team or the health care system itself, or any action on the part of others that is prejudicial to the client's best interests. To function effectively in the role, the nurse should be fully aware of the state laws governing practice in the health care field and the employing institution's policies and procedures in relation to incompetent, unethical, or illegal practice.

3.2 INITIAL ACTION

When the nurse is aware of inappropriate or questionable conduct in the provision of health care, concern should be expressed to the person carrying out the questionable practice and attention called to the possible detrimental effect upon the client's welfare. When factors in the health care delivery system threaten the welfare of the client, similar action should be directed to the responsible administrative person. If indicated, the practice should then be reported to the appropriate authority within the institution, agency, or larger system. There should be an established mechanism for the reporting and handling of incompetent, unethical, or illegal practice within the employment setting so that such reporting can go through official channels and be done without fear of reprisal. The nurse should be knowledgeable about the mechanism and be prepared to utilize it if necessary. When questions are raised about the appropriateness of behaviors of individual practitioners or practices of health care systems, documentation of the observed behavior or practice must be provided in writing to the appropriate authorities. Local units of the professional association should be prepared to provide assistance and support in reporting procedures.

3.3 FOLLOW-UP ACTION

When incompetent, unethical, or illegal practice on the part of anyone concerned with the client's care is not corrected within the employment setting and continues to jeopardize the client's care and safety, additional steps need to be taken. The problem should be reported to other appropriate authorities such as the practice committees of the appropriate professional organizations or the legally constituted bodies concerned with licensing of specific categories of health workers or professional practitioners. Some situations may warrant the concern and involvement of all these groups. Reporting should be both factual and objective.

3.4 PEER REVIEW

In addition to the role of advocate, the nurse should participate in the planning, establishment, and implementation of other activities or procedures which serve to safeguard clients. Duly constituted peer review activities in employment agencies directed toward the improvement of practice are one example. This ongoing method of review is based on objective criteria, it includes a mechanism for making recommendations to administrators for correction of deficiencies, it facilitates the improvement of delivery services, and it promotes the health, welfare, and safety of clients.

4. THE NURSE ASSUMES RESPONSIBILITY AND ACCOUNTABILITY FOR INDIVIDUAL NURSING JUDGMENTS AND ACTIONS.

4.1 ACCEPTANCE OF RESPONSIBILITY AND ACCOUNTABILITY

The recipients of professional nursing services are entitled to high quality nursing care. Individual professional licensure is the protective mechanism legislated by the public to ensure basic and minimum competencies of the professional nurse. Beyond that, society has accorded to the nursing profession the right to regulate its own practice. The regulation and control of nursing practice by nurses demands that individual professional practitioners of nursing bear primary responsibility for the nursing care clients receive and be individually accountable for their practice.

4.2 RESPONSIBILITY

Responsibility refers to the scope of functions and duties associated with a particular role assumed by the nurse. As nursing assumes functions, these functions become part of the responsibilities or expectations of performance of nurses. Areas of responsibilities expected of nurses include: data collection and assessment of the health status of the client; determination of the nursing care plan directed toward designated goals; evaluation of the effectiveness of nursing care in achieving the goals of care; and subsequent reassessment and revision of the nursing care plan as defined in the ANA Standards of Nursing Practice. By assuming these responsibilities, the nurse is held accountable for them.

4.3 ACCOUNTABILITY

Accountability refers to being answerable to someone for something one has done. It means providing an explanation to self, to the client, to the employing agency, and to the nursing profession. Over and above the obligations such accountability imposes on the individual nurse, there is also a liability dimension to accountability. The nurse may be called to account to be held legally responsible for judgments exercised and actions taken in the course of nursing practice. Neither physician's prescriptions nor the employing agency's policies relieve the nurse of ethical or legal accountability for actions taken and judgments made. Accountability, therefore, requires evaluation of the effectiveness of one's performance of nursing responsibilities.

4.4 EVALUATION OF PERFORMANCE

Self-evaluation. The nurse engaged in ongoing evaluation of individual clinical competence, decision-making abilities, and professional judgments. The nurse also engages in activities that will improve current practice. Self-evaluation carries with it the responsibility for the continuous improvement of one's nursing practice.

Evaluation by peers. Evaluation of one's performance by peers is a hallmark of professionalism, and it is primarily through this mechanism that the profession is held accountable to society. The nurse must be willing to have practice reviewed and evaluated by peers. Guidelines for evaluating the appropriateness, effectiveness, and efficiency of nursing practice are emerging in the form of revised and updated nurse practice acts, ANA's Standards of Nursing Practice, and other quality assurance mechanisms. Participation in the development of objective criteria for evaluation that provide valid and reliable data is the responsibility of each nurse.

5. THE NURSE MAINTAINS COMPETENCE IN NURSING.

5.1 PERSONAL RESPONSIBILITY FOR COMPETENCE

Nursing is concerned with the welfare of human beings, and the nature of nursing is such that inadequate or incompetent practice may jeopardize the client. Therefore, it is the personal responsibility and must be the personal commitment of each individual nurse to maintain competence in practice throughout a professional career. This represents one way in which the nurse fulfills accountability to clients.

5.2 MEASUREMENT OF COMPETENCE IN NURSING PRACTICE

Competence is a relative term, and an individual's competence in any field may be diminished or otherwise affected by the passage of time and the emergence of new knowledge. This means that for the client's optimum well-being and for the nurse's own professional development, nursing care should reflect and incorporate new techniques and knowledge in health care as these develop and especially as they relate to the nurse's particular field of practice.

Measures of competence are developing; they include peer review criteria, outcome criteria, and ANA's program for certification.

5.3 CONTINUING EDUCATION FOR CONTINUING COMPETENCE

Nursing knowledge, like that in the other health disciplines, is rendered rapidly obsolete by mounting technological advances and scientific discoveries, changing concepts and patterns in the provision of health services, and the increasing complexity of nursing responsibilities. The nurse, therefore, should be aware of the need for continuous updating and expansion of the body of knowledge on which practice is based and should keep knowledge and skills current. The nurse should assess personal learning needs, should be active in finding appropriate resources, and should be skilled in self-directed learning. Such continuing education is the key to maintenance of individual competence.

5.4 INTRAPROFESSIONAL RESPONSIBILITY FOR COMPETENCE IN NURSING CARE

All nurses, be they practitioners, educators, administrators, or researchers, share responsibility for quality nursing care. Therefore all nurses need thorough knowledge of the current scope of professional nursing practice. Advances in theory and practice made by one professional must be disseminated to colleagues. Since individual competencies vary in relation to educational preparation, experience, client population and setting, when necessary, nurses should refer clients to and/or consult with other nurses with expertise and recognized competencies, e.g. certified nurses and clinical specialists.

6. THE NURSE EXERCISES INFORMED JUDGMENT AND USES INDIVIDUAL COMPETENCE AND QUALIFICATIONS AS CRITERIA IN SEEKING CONSULTATION, ACCEPTING RESPONSIBILITIES, AND DELEGATING NURSING ACTIVITIES TO OTHERS.

6.1 CHANGING FUNCTIONS

Because of the increased complexity of health care, changing patterns in the delivery of health services, continuing shortages in skilled health manpower, and the development acceptance of evolving nursing roles, nurses are being requested or expected to carry out functions that have formerly been performed by physicians. In turn, nurses are assigning some nursing functions to variously prepared ancillary personnel. In this gradual shift of functions, as the scope of practice of each profession changes, the nurse must exercise judgment in seeking consultation, accepting responsibilities, and assigning responsibilities to others to ensure that clients receive quality care at all times.

6.2 JOINT POLICY STATEMENTS

Nurse practice acts are usually expressed in broad and general language in order to provide the necessary freedom for interpretation of the law so that future developments, new knowledge, and changing roles will not necessitate constant revision of the law. The nurse must not engage in practice prohibited by law or delegate to others activities prohibited by practice acts of other health care personnel or by other laws. Recognition by nurses of the need for a more definitive delineation of roles and responsibilities, however, has resulted in collaborative efforts to develop joint policy statements. These statements may involve other health care providers or associations and usually specify the functions that are agreed upon as appropriate and proper for the nurse to perform. Such statements represent a body of expert judgment that can be used as authority where responsibilities are not definitively outlined by legal statute.

6.3 SEEKING CONSULTATION

The provision of health and illness care to clients is a complex process that requires a wide range of knowledge and skills. Interdisciplinary team effort with shared responsibility is the most effective approach to provision of total health services. Nurses, whether practicing in clearly defined or new and emerging roles, must be aware of their own individual competencies. When the needs of the client are beyond the qualifications and competencies of the nurse, consultation must be sought from qualified nurses or other appropriate sources.

Discretion must be exercised by the nurse before intervening in diagnostic or therapeutic matters that are not recognized by the nursing profession as established nursing practice. Such discretion should be based on education, experience, legal parameters, and professional guidelines and policies.

6.4 ACCEPTING RESPONSIBILITIES OR DELEGATING ACTIVITIES

The nurse should look to mutually agreed upon policy statements for guidance and direction; but even where such statements exist, personal competence should be carefully assessed before accepting responsibility or delegating activities. Decisions in this area call for knowledge of and adherence to joint policy statements and the laws regulating medical and nursing practice as well as for the exercise of informed nursing judgments.

6.5 ACCEPTING RESPONSIBILITY

If the nurse does not feel personally competent or adequately prepared to carry out a specific function, the nurse has the right and responsibility to refuse. In so doing, both the client and the nurse are protected. The reverse is also true. The nurse should not accept delegated responsibilities that do not utilize nursing skill or competencies or that prevent the provision of needed nursing care to clients. Inasmuch as the nurse is responsible for the client's total nursing care, the nurse must also assess individual competence in assigning selected components of that care to other nursing service personnel. The nurse should not delegate to any member of the nursing team a function for which that person is not prepared or qualified to perform.

7. THE NURSE PARTICIPATES IN ACTIVITIES THAT CONTRIBUTE TO THE ONGOING DEVELOPMENT OF THE PROFESSION'S BODY OF KNOWLEDGE.

7.1 THE NURSE AND RESEARCH

Every profession must engage in systematic inquiry to identify, verify, and continually enlarge the body of knowledge which forms the foundations for its practice. A unique body of verified knowledge provides both framework and direction for the profession in all of its activities and for the practitioner in the provision of nursing care. The accrual of knowledge promotes the advancement of practice and with it the well-being of the profession's clients. Ongoing research is thus indispensable to the full discharge of a profession's obligations to society. Each nurse has a role in this area of professional activity, whether involved as an investigator in the furthering of knowledge, as a participant in research, or as a user of research results.

7.2 GENERAL GUIDELINES FOR PARTICIPATING IN RESEARCH

Before participating in research the nurse has an obligation:

1. To ascertain that the study design has been approved by an appropriate body.
2. To obtain information about the intent and the nature of the research.
3. To determine whether the research is consistent with professional goals.

Research involving human subjects should be conducted only by scientifically qualified persons or under such supervision. The nurse who participates in research in any capacity should be fully informed about both nurse and client rights and responsibilities as set forth in the publication *Human Rights Guidelines for Nurses in Clinical and Other Research* prepared by the ANA Commission on Nursing Research.

7.3 THE PROTECTION OF HUMAN RIGHTS IN RESEARCH

The individual rights valued by society and by the nursing profession have been fully outlined and discussed in *Human Rights Guidelines for Nurses in Clinical and Other Research;* namely, the right to freedom from intrinsic risks of injury and the rights of privacy and dignity. Inherent in these rights is respect for each individual to exercise self-determination, to choose to participate, to have full information, to terminate participation without penalty.

It is the duty of both the investigator and the nurse participating in research to maintain vigilance in protecting the life, health, and privacy of human subjects from unanticipated as well as anticipated risks. The subjects' integrity, privacy, and rights must be especially safeguarded if they are unable to protect themselves because of incapacity or because they are in a dependent relationship to the investigator. The investigation should be discontinued if its continuance might be harmful to the subject.

7.4 THE PRACTITIONER'S RIGHTS AND RESPONSIBILITIES IN RESEARCH

Practitioners of nursing providing care to clients who serve as human subjects for research have a special need to clearly understand in advance how the research can be expected to affect treatment and their own moral and legal responsibilities to clients. Here, as in other problematic situations, the practitioner has the right not to participate or to withdraw under the circumstances described in paragraph 1.4 of this document. More detailed guidance about the rights and responsibilities of nurses in relation to research activities may be found in *Human Rights Guidelines for Nurses in Clinical and Other Research.*

8. THE NURSE PARTICIPATES IN THE PROFESSION'S EFFORTS TO IMPLEMENT AND IMPROVE STANDARDS OF NURSING.

8.1 RESPONSIBILITY TO THE PUBLIC

Nursing has the responsibility to admit to the profession only those who have demonstrated a capacity for those competencies believed essential to the practice of nursing. Areas of concern for nursing competence should include adequate performance of nursing skills, academic achievement, humanitarian concern for others, acceptance of responsibility for individual actions, and the desire to improve nursing practice. Nurses involved in the evaluation of student attainment carry a primary responsibility for ensuring that the profession's obligation to the public relative to entry qualifications for practice are met.

The nursing profession exists to give assistance to those persons needing nursing care. Standards of nursing practice provide guidance for the delivery of quality nursing care and are a means for evaluating that care received by clients. The nurse has a responsibility to the public for personally implementing and maintaining optimal standards.

8.2 RESPONSIBILITY TO THE DISCIPLINE

The professional practice of nursing is founded on an understanding and application of a body of knowledge reflected in its standards. As the profession's organization for nurses, ANA has adopted standards for nursing practice, nursing service, and nursing education. The nurse has the responsibility to monitor these standards in everyday practice and through voluntary participation in the profession's ongoing efforts to implement and improve standards at the national, state, and local levels.

8.3 RESPONSIBILITY TO NURSING STUDENTS

The future of nursing rests with new recruits to the profession. Nursing has a responsibility to maintain optimal standards of nursing practice and education in schools of nursing and/or wherever students engage in learning activity. This places a particular responsibility on all nurses whose services are concerned with the educational process.

9. THE NURSE PARTICIPATES IN THE PROFESSION'S EFFORTS TO ESTABLISH AND MAINTAIN CONDITIONS OF EMPLOYMENT CONDUCIVE TO HIGH QUALITY NURSING CARE.

9.1 RESPONSIBILITY FOR CONDITIONS OF EMPLOYMENT

The nurse must be concerned with conditions of economic and general welfare within the profession. These are important determinants in the recruitment and retention of well-qualified personnel and in assuring that each practitioner has the opportunity to function optimally.

The provision of high quality nursing care is the responsibility of both the individual nurse and the nursing profession. Professional autonomy and self-regulation in the control of conditions of practice are necessary to implement standards of practice as established by organized nursing.

9.2 COLLECTIVE ACTION

Defining and controlling the quality of nursing care provided to the client is most effectively accomplished through collective action. Collective action may include assistance and representation from the professional association in negotiations with employers to achieve employment conditions in which the professional standards of practice can be implemented and which are commensurate with the qualifications, functions, and responsibilities of the nurse. The Economic and General Welfare program of the professional association is the appropriate channel through which the nurse can work constructively, ethically, and with professional dignity. This program, encompassing commitment to the principle of collective bargaining, promotes the right and responsibility of the individual nurse to participate in determining the terms and conditions of employment conducive to high quality nursing practice.

9.3 INDIVIDUAL ACTION

A nurse may enter into an agreement with individuals or organizations to provide health care, provided that the agreement is in accordance with the Standards of Nursing Practice of the American Nurses' Association and the nurse practice law of the state and provided that the agreement does not permit or compel practices which are in violation of this Code.

10. THE NURSE PARTICIPATES IN THE PROFESSION'S EFFORT TO PROTECT THE PUBLIC FROM MISINFORMATION AND MISREPRESENTATION AND TO MAINTAIN THE INTEGRITY OF NURSING.

10.1 ADVERTISING SERVICES

A nurse may make factual statements that indicate availability of services through means that are in dignified form, such as:

> A professional card identifying the nurse by name and title, giving address, telephone number, and other pertinent data.
>
> Listing name, title, and brief biography in reputable directories and reputable professional publications. Such published data may include the following: Name, address, phone, field of practice or concentrates; date and place of birth; schools attended, with dates of graduation, degrees, and other scholastic distinctions; offices held; public or professional honors; teaching positions; publications; memberships and activities in professional societies; licenses; names and addresses of references.

A nurse shall not use any form of public or professional communication to make self-laudatory statements of claims that are false, fraudulent, misleading, deceptive, or unfair.

10.2 USE OF TITLES AND SYMBOLS

The right to use the title "Registered Nurse" is granted by state governments through licensure by examination for the protection of the public. Use of that title carries with it the responsibility to act in the public interest. The nurse may use the title "R.N." and symbols of academic degrees or other earned or honorary professional symbols of recognition in all ways that are legal and appropriate. The title and other symbols of the profession should not be used, however, for personal benefit by the nurse or by those who may seek to exploit them for other purposes.

10.3 ENDORSEMENT OF COMMERCIAL PRODUCTS OR SERVICES

The nurse does not give or imply endorsement to advertising, promotion, or sale of commercial products or services because this may be interpreted as reflecting the opinion or judgment of the profession as a whole. Since it is a nursing responsibility to engage in health teaching and to advise clients on matters relating to their health, it is not unethical for the nurse to utilize knowledge of specific services and/or products in advising individual clients. In the course of providing information or education to clients or other practitioners about commercial products or services, however, a variety of similar products or services should be offered or described so that the client or practitioner can make an informed choice.

10.4 PROTECTING THE CLIENT FROM HARMFUL PRODUCTS

It is the responsibility of the nurse to advise clients against the use of dangerous products. This is seen as discharge of nursing functions when undertaken in the best interest of the client.

10.5 REPORTING INFRACTIONS

Not only should the nurse personally adhere to the above principles, but alertness to any instances of their violation by others should be maintained. The nurse should report promptly, through appropriate channels, any advertisement or commercial which involves a nurse, implies involvement, or in any way suggests nursing endorsement of a commercial product, service, or enterprise. The nurse who knowingly becomes involved in such unethical activities negates professional responsibility for personal gain, and jeopardizes the public confidence and trust in the nursing profession that have been created by generations of nurses working together in the public interest.

11. THE NURSE COLLABORATES WITH MEMBERS OF THE HEALTH PROFESSIONS AND OTHER CITIZENS IN PROMOTING COMMUNITY AND NATIONAL EFFORTS TO MEET THE HEALTH NEEDS OF THE PUBLIC.

11.1 QUALITY HEALTH CARE AS A RIGHT

Quality health care is mandated as a right to all citizens. Availability and accessibility to quality health services for all citizens require collaborative planning by health providers and consumers at both the local and national level. Nursing care is an integral part of quality heath care, and nurses have a responsibility to help ensure that citizens' rights to health care are met.

11.2 RESPONSIBILITY TO THE CONSUMER OF HEALTH CARE

The nurse is a member of the largest group of health providers, and therefore the philosophies and goals of the nursing profession should have a significant impact on the consumer of health care. An effective way of ensuring that nurses' views regarding health care and nursing service are represented is by involvement of nurses in political decision making.

11.3 RELATIONSHIPS WITH OTHER DISCIPLINES

The complexity of the delivery of health care service demands an interdisciplinary approach to delivery of health services as well as strong support from allied health occupations. The nurse should actively seek to promote collaboration needed for ensuring the quality of health services to all persons.

11.4 RELATIONSHIP WITH MEDICINE

The interdependent relationship of the nursing and medical professions requires collaboration around the need of the client. The evolving role of the nurse in the health delivery system requires joint practice as colleagues, deliberations in determining functional relationships, and differentiating areas of practice between the two professions.

11.5 CONFLICT OF INTEREST

Nurses who provide public service and who have financial or other interests in health care facilities or services should avoid a conflict of interest by refraining from casting a vote on any deliberation affecting the public's health care needs in those areas.

READING E

Rcn CODE OF PROFESSIONAL CONDUCT—A DISCUSSION DOCUMENT

TEXT

I Introduction

The profession of nursing has a commitment which is shared with other health care professions to promote optimal standards of health, combat disease and disability and alleviate suffering. A code of professional conduct is required in order to make explicit those moral standards which should guide professional decisions in these matters, and in order to encourage responsible moral decision making throughout the profession. It is recognized that no code can do justice to every individual case and therefore that any set of principles must remain constantly open to discussion both within the nursing profession and outside it.

DISCUSSION

I The starting point of this code is the recognition that nursing is now a profession in its own right, with all the responsibility which that entails. It shares with other professions—notably medicine and social work—the goal of improving the health prospects of all members of that society which grants it the right to practice. Because ideas about health goals vary from individual to individual, and because nurses have considerable influence (and on occasion power) over patients or clients whose needs and handicaps often render them especially vulnerable, a code of conduct is needed to provide guidelines for professional practice. Such a code ought to be continuously developed and refined by sustained discussion among nurses themselves, and by consultation between nurses and those who can speak for other professions and for the general public.

Codes are never a substitute for personal moral integrity, and they can often be hardened into legal formulae. It must therefore be stressed that the purpose of this code is not to devise grounds for disciplinary proceedings (or any similar purpose), but rather to provide a clear and comprehensive document for further discussion, particularly during periods of professional training.

II Responsibility to Patients or Clients

The primary responsibility of nurses is to protect and enhance the wellbeing and dignity of each individual person in their care. As members of professional teams nurses should recognize and accept responsibility for the total effects of nursing and medical care on individuals. This responsibility is in no way affected by the type of origin of the person's need or illness or by his age, sex, mental status, social class, ethnic origins, nationality or personal beliefs. Therefore it follows that:

(1) Nursing care should be directed towards the preservation, or restoration, as far as is possible, of a person's ability to function normally and independently within his own chosen environment.

(2) Discrimination against particular individuals, for whatever reason, should never be tolerated.

II

(1) As a form of social occupation nursing serves several ends: it provides paid employment to a large section of society; it gives individuals a sense of intellectual achievement and job satisfaction; and it offers congenial and rewarding inter- and intra-professional relationships. But none of these should take precedence over the primary end of nursing, which is to enable people to live their own lives as fully and freely as possible by providing professional counsel and care according to particular needs.

(2) Entering the nursing profession involves a commitment to the service of persons, each of whom merits individual respect. At times nurses may have prejudices against patients or clients because they consider that they are largely responsible for their own misfortune or because they cannot feel any sympathy for their particular form of distress. But the adoption of a professional attitude requires that all those who need nursing care should receive it without discrimination.

No group of patients or clients should be regarded as unworthy or undeserving of professional concern.

(3) During episodes of illness the autonomy of patients should be maintained throughout treatment, restrictions being imposed only when these are demonstrably necessary for their own wellbeing, or for the safety of others; and the active participation of patients in their own treatment should be facilitated by means of open and sensitive communication.

(3) Nurses share in responsibility for the effect of the multidisciplinary treatment methods of modern medicine on personal health and freedom. In particular, the routines of hospitals and health institutions and other organizational structures may unnecessarily remove the dignity and independence of patients, thereby diminishing their overall health prospects. In view of this a fundamental aspect of the nurse's responsibility to the patient can be seen as the maintenance and restoration of personal autonomy. This is principally achieved by skilled nursing care of each individual, with an understanding of the context of his illness or disability and with careful attention being paid to communication with him, especially during periods of anxiety. In this context it should be noted that the best source of information about the patient is usually the patient himself and that regular and relaxed discussions with relatives can increase the nurse's understanding of the patient's circumstances and of possible ways in which he can be helped to achieve an optimal level of living. It is recognized that dealing with violent or potentially violent patients raises particularly difficult problems in relation to restraint and patients' freedom. It is essential that clear guidelines are given to all those who have such patients in their care to ensure that prejudice and mutual fear between patients and staff do not worsen the situation. (See the guidelines offered by the DHSS on the basis of joint advice from the Rcn and the Royal College of Psychiatrists—The Management of Violent or Potentially Violent Hospital Patients. Hc(76)11).

(4) Measures which jeopardize the safety of patients, such as unnecessary treatments, hazardous experimental procedures and the withdrawal of professional services during employment disputes, should be actively opposed by the profession as a whole.

(4) Actions which betray people's confidence in the professional integrity of nurses diminish the ability of the profession to be of help. For this reason the nursing profession should be clearly seen to be opposed to exploitation of vulnerability, for example: Treatment and Experimentation—inappropriate treatment, risky experimentation or experimentation without proper consent; or Industrial Action—the removal of professional services which put patients at risk.

Although choice of treatments and the initiation of clinical research projects is usually solely a medical responsibility, nurses have the right and the duty to express opinions about the effect of such procedures on the patients under their care. (For instance a nurse may question whether the dignity of a dying patient is being respected by procedures employed to delay death; and the design of an experiment involving discomfort or risk to patients may be questioned by nurses asked to co-operate in the experiment.)

Nurses are entitled to equitable wages and conditions of employment and should be free to enter into appropriate negotiations with their employers. But since seriously ill people are in no position to protect themselves when professional aid is withdrawn, disruption of services by strike action and threats to do so contravene the nurse's commitment to service of patients and should be publicly opposed, whether the action is carried out by nurses or by other professions and occupations involved in health care.

(5) Information about patients or clients should be treated with the utmost confidence and respect, and should not be divulged to persons outwith the primary care or treat-

(5) In unusual circumstances it may be necessary to disclose confidential information for the wellbeing of the patient or others in the nurse's care, but this should never be done without full consultation with relatives and with medical and nursing colleagues; and when-

ment team without the person's consent, except in exceptional circumstances.

ever possible the patient should be told why such a disclosure was felt to be necessary.

III Responsibility for Professional Standards

The professional authority of nurses is based upon their training and experience in day to day care of ill persons at home or in hospital; and in the enhancement of positive health in the community at large. All members of the nursing profession have a responsibility to continue to develop their knowledge and skill in these matters.

III This claim to professional status implies that nurses have particular forms of knowledge and skill in health care which are not shared by other professions and which thereby give them the authority to institute nursing procedures and make decisions and recommendations about correct nursing care.

This claim must be substantiated by the profession as a whole through the establishment of training procedures and the maintenance of competence at all levels within the profession and by continued research into new and improved methods of nursing care.

Individual nurses have the responsibility to be self-critical of their professional performance and to seek to adapt it to changing needs and new techniques of care.

IV Responsibility to Colleagues

In general, relationships with colleagues in nursing and in other health care professions should be determined according to what will maximize the benefit of those in their care.

IV The goal of 'whole person treatment' determines how nurses should relate professionally to their fellow nurses and to members of other health care professions. It is assumed that the more there is co-operation and communication between the different people caring for the patient, the more the patient's needs are likely to be understood and catered for. (As noted in the previous section, the patient himself has also a great deal to contribute to such full understanding, as do his relatives.)

(1) Professional relationships between

(1) The nursing 'hierarchy' can be seen to be necessary to ensure that

nurses should be regulated according to the level of knowledge, experience and skill of each nurse. Clear chains of command should be established to deal with emergency situations, but except in such situations, free discussion of the reasons for established procedures should be encouraged at all levels.

(2) Professional relationships between nurses and doctors should be regulated according to the particular expertise of each profession. In the case of medical treatments nurses are under an obligation to carry out a doctor's instructions except where they have a good reason to believe that harm will be caused to the patient by so doing. In cases in which nurses' continuous contact with the patient has given them a different insight into the patient's medical needs, they are under moral obligation to communicate this to the doctor in charge of the case. Nurses should support the multi-disciplinary case-conference approach to the treatment decisions, and should improve their ability to participate actively in such conferences.

(3) Professional relationships between nurses and members of other health care

decisions are taken by those who should have the requisite knowledge and experience, but on the other hand junior members of staff can often bring fresh insights about patients or be more successful in gaining the patient's confidence. For this reason an atmosphere of friendly questioning and discussion between staff at different levels can improve the quality of care as well as making nurse education more effective. (Obviously clear lines of authority are needed for situations in which rapid decisions have to be made.)

(2) Nurses are not trained to diagnose illness or to prescribe medical treatment. They must therefore normally carry out doctors' instructions in these matters and help maintain the patient's confidence in his medical advisors. But nurses are in a unique position to observe the condition of the patient at all hours of day and night and have received basic instruction in drug dosages, effects of treatment, etc. For this reason they are morally obligated to question medical instructions which they believe will cause the patient harm or unnecessary distress (see Section II above) even though they may fear adverse effects on their career from doing so. Ideally, however, this should not entail a confrontation between doctor and nurse, but should arise naturally in the context of ongoing inter-professional discussions in case conferences. Part of the professional training of nurses should prepare them to take part in such conferences from their own professional standpoint.

(3) In the case of other professions which may have contact with patients or clients (e.g. paramedical professions, social workers,

professions should be based upon respect for each other's area of expertise and on the desire to gain a fuller understanding of the patient's or client's needs. Procedures should be established for regular interprofessional consultations.

hospital chaplains and other clergy) nurses should be concerned to establish relationships of trust. This should promote a mutual understanding of professional roles enabling the patient/client to derive maximum benefit from the work of the caring team.

V Professional Responsibility and Personal Responsibility

As citizens of a state and as private individuals nurses should defend and actively pursue those moral values to which their profession is committed, namely, individual autonomy, parity of treatment and the pursuit of health. In some circumstances this may require protest against, and opposition to, social and political conditions which are detrimental to human wellbeing; and in others, the altering of personal habits which set a poor example in health care. In all other respects nurses have the right to regulate their private lives according to their own standards of morality, provided their style of life does not cast doubts on the integrity and trustworthiness of their profession.

V Because nursing finds its origins partly in religious orders, there may be unrealistic expectations both within the profession and amongst the general public about the degree of personal dedication to which modern nurses should aspire. Like other professionals, nurses have the right to conduct their private lives without undue interference from colleagues or employers. Also like other professionals, however, the choice of a personal service career commits the nurse to certain moral views. Nurses cannot strive to alleviate disease and suffering without becoming aware of the social circumstances which bring it about or which inhibit the provision of effective remedies. It follows that nurses should be concerned with political and social issues, whenever these are relevant to the prevention of disease or the delivery of health care. Similarly in the sphere of personal conduct, nurses should strive to 'practice what they preach' to avoid personal habits which are known to be detrimental to health. (For example, doctors and nurses are particularly at risk for drug and alcohol addiction—a factor which seems to demand closer supportive attention from their respective professions.)

In addition to setting a good example in healthy styles of life, nurses need to inspire confidence in patients in order to be able to help them fully. This does not imply 'angelic' purity of life—merely the following of standards of honesty and of moral seriousness which would be expected from any member of society who has responsibility for the welfare of others.

READING F

HUMAN RIGHTS GUIDELINES FOR NURSES IN CLINICAL AND OTHER RESEARCH

AMERICAN NURSES' ASSOCIATION

INTRODUCTION

The American Nurses' Association in establishing a Commission on Nursing Research publicly reaffirmed the nursing profession's obligation to support the advancement of scientific knowledge toward the achievement of improved nursing practice and better patient care. In taking this step the organization accepted a commitment to support two sets of human rights. One set is concerned with the rights of qualified nurses (those with research preparation) to engage in research and to have access to resources necessary for implementing scientific investigations. The other deals with the human rights of all persons who are recipients of health care services or are participants in research performed by investigators whose studies impinge on the patient care provided by nurses. The need for the establishment of human rights guidelines for nurses came as a result of social and technical changes that altered nursing and nursing practice.

In the twentieth century, nurses engage in a variety of activities that impinge upon the rights of other human beings. Some nurses participate as investigators in organized research utilizing animals or human beings as subjects of study. Other nurses are employed in work settings in which clinical medical activities and technical procedures have moved into the domain of the unusual or extraordinary. Probably the majority of nurses continue to perform activities that are usual and expected according to the norms of accepted practice, but increasingly the borderline between usual and expected and "experimental" clinical practices is becoming blurred. As the scope of nursing practice has increased in complexity, nursing as a profession has had an increased concern with the human rights of all

---

persons who are recipients of nursing services or are participants in clinical research.

The relationship of trust between patient and nurse has always been an essential element of the professional code of ethics. In research, the relationship of trust between subject and investigator requires that the investigator assumes special obligations to safeguard the subject in several ways. The subject needs to be assured that his rights will not be violated without his voluntary and informed consent. Secondly, the investigator guarantees that no risk, discomfort, invasion of privacy, or threat to personal dignity beyond that initially stated in describing the subject's role in the study will be imposed without further permission being obtained. Finally, the subject is assured that if he does not wish to participate in the study, he will neither be subjected to harrassment nor will the quality of his care be influenced by this decision.

The members of the ANA Commission on Nursing Research believe that each individual has the right of self-determination concerning what will be done to his person. The members also believe that each practitioner of nursing has an obligation to endorse and support self-determination as a moral and legal right of the individual. The responsibilities attendant to safeguarding the rights of other people must be freely accepted by nurses whether their roles be practitioners, educators, or researchers.

Changing Scope of Responsibility

The scope of nurses' responsibilities in relation to human rights issues has gradually extended in response to continued professional dialogue, public debate, and legal testing of individual cases. Some substantive areas such as death and dying, population control, genetic engineering, and manipulation of behavior are emerging already as significant social issues and problems in nursing practice. Consequent ramifications regarding "informed consent" by the individual involve both practitioners and researchers when invasion of privacy, dehumanization, and risk are potentially present. Furthermore, health as a national resource or public good involves new social and scientific dimensions when decisions regarding the use of scarce resources such as hemodialysis and transplants must be made.

The ethical standards and guidelines established at any given time by the nursing profession need to be sufficiently flexible to be applicable to new issues as they emerge under the influence of science or technology. Clear standards and flexible guidelines are essential if science and social values are to change and develop together in relative harmony rather than in conflict. To be effective such guidelines must also clearly delineate and specify the circumstances under which they apply. The guidelines that follow attempt to specify several important entities: the type of activities that are involved; the rights that are to be protected; the persons to be safeguarded; and mechanisms necessary to ensure that protection is adequate.

ETHICAL GUIDELINES

Nursing Activities and Ethical Issues

The need for protection of human rights potentially involves all activities that go beyond the established and accepted practices of the professional group involved. In health care practice, the need for protection of human rights is of singular importance for any and all activities when the focus is not specifically directed toward meeting the needs of the individual patient or subject. The development and refinement of scientific knowledge in nursing will increasingly involve nurses in clinical investigations with an emphasis on furthering knowledge rather than specifically on meeting patients' needs. Other nurses in their roles as practitioners in hospitals and other institutional settings can find themselves engaged in clinical research developed and implemented by practitioners in other fields. In both cases, ethical concerns about the potential violations of human rights become crucial whenever new and untried techniques and procedures are to be used and when the probable outcomes are unknown or doubtful.

Whenever nurses perform activities that are components of clinical research (whether directed by physicians, nurses, or other investigators), the need for protection of human rights must extend to the practitioners who are expected to participate in new and untried practices as well as to the subjects who are recipients of them. The concept of informed consent applies not only to subjects *per se* but also to any workers who are expected as part of their daily work to implement activities that potentially or actually carry risk for others or have uncertain outcomes.

Implementation of this guideline implies the need for written statements about conditions of employment and any special expectations about work performance above and beyond that usually expected of a person occupying the position of nurse. In advance of such employment, nurses need to know if they will be expected to provide medicines, treatments, and other procedures as part of double blind investigations.

They need to know in advance if the work requires them to function as data-collectors for research in addition to their roles as nurses engaged in the delivery of patient care services. Conditions of employment must also provide for the option of not participating in clinical research if these work expectations are not spelled out in advance of employment.

Stated in a more general way, conditions of employment in settings in which clinical and/or other research is in progress need to be spelled out in detail for all potential workers. As a corollary, it follows that anyone employed in work that carries the potential of risk to others needs to be advised as to the types of risks involved, the ways of recognizing when risk is present, and the proper actions to take to counteract harmful effects and unnecessary danger.

Human Rights

Right to Freedom from Intrinsic Risk of Injury

In situations in which the nature of the activities or research design exposes an individual to increased possibility of emotional, social, or physical injury, the degree of risk needs to be estimated and specified by the principal investigator or his designate. It is incumbent upon all practitioners to recognize that risk is potentially present in all situations when novel and untried procedures are involved and there is little if any data upon which to predict outcomes. The primary problem faced by the investigator or practitioner is prediction of the extent of risk to the individual in comparison to the potential clinical benefit to him and/or the humanitarian importance of the knowledge to be gained.

In all instances, the prospective subject must be given all relevant information prior to participation in activities that go beyond established and accepted procedures necessary to meet his personal needs. By virtue of their calling, practitioners in the health professions seek to protect individuals under their care from arbitrary physical or mental suffering. Nurses must be increasingly vigilant in their concern for subjects and patients who by reason of their situation and/or illness are not able to protect themselves effectively from externally imposed threat or injury. They must also be sensitive to the tendency toward exploitation of "captive" populations such as students, patients in institutions, and prisoners.

Right of Privacy and Dignity

Human beings vary in their values and judgments about what is considered invasion of privacy and a threat to dignity through demeaning or dehumanizing conditions. The investigator cannot presume to decide for the other person on this matter of privacy and dignity. Consequently all proposals, investigative instruments, protocols, and techniques to be used in the particular activities need to be specified and discussed with the prospective subject and with any workers who are expected to participate in the activity as subjects, as data-collectors, or as both.

Consideration must be given to the development of safeguards such that no unanticipated physical, psychological, or social disadvantage accrues to subjects either during the study or as a result of dissemination of the findings. If the subject agrees voluntarily to share certain specific information about himself which he may or may not choose to divulge to others in a different context, then the investigator must provide assurance that the subject's anonymity will be protected. Specific prior consent must be obtained whenever the plan of a study or a report of findings sacrifices subject anonymity or confidentiality.

Special mechanisms for safeguarding the confidentiality of information must be developed whenever the information will not always remain under the control of the investigator. Potentially demeaning or dehumanizing conditions merit special consideration from both practitioners and investigators inasmuch as they are in many instances difficult to specify and to protect against. Health care practitioners need to be aware that violations involving human dignity have many potential long range repercussions when significant values of the individual are involved.

Subjects

The persons for whom human rights guidelines apply include all individuals involved in the activities described before. When activities are supported either directly or indirectly by government and other funding resources, the persons to whom these guidelines apply include the following groups: patients; outpatients; donors of organs, tissues, and services; informants; normal volunteers including students; and volunteers in groups with limited civil freedom. The latter classification refers to prisoners, residents or clients in institutions for the mentally ill and mentally retarded, and persons subject to military discipline, all of whom tend easily to fall into the class of captive audience and population vulnerable to exploitation.

The choice of minors and groups with limited civil freedom as research subjects can be justified, in most instances, only if there are benefits that will accrue in the future to them or to others in similar situations or classes. Strict standards governing the use of minors and other groups (including the unborn and the dead) lacking the capacity to give informed consent are being established with increasing frequency by various government statutes and regulations.

Society's Obligation and the Public Good

In a democratic society the rights of the individual are of necessity counterbalanced by actions and activities designed for the common good of collective man. Established public health practices such as the immunization of children against diphtheria and pertussis and the chlorination of public water supplies to prevent epidemics of water-borne disease are examples of societal actions in which personal rights gave way to collective rights for the benefit of society as a whole. These and many other public health practices came into being as a result of research seeking ways to treat and control disease.

Advancement of knowledge about health and health-promoting practices is also of value to society as a whole. So too is knowledge about patient responses and adaptations to illness and the effects of different nursing interventions on these responses and adaptations. Just as nurses have an obligation to protect the human rights of patients, so do they also have an obligation to support the accrual of knowledge that broadens the scientific underpinnings of nursing practice and the delivery of nursing services. Professional responsibility includes a recognition that research by qualified nurses is a resource in need of support and encouragement.

MECHANISMS FOR PROTECTION OF RIGHTS

Assurance—Informed Consent

To safeguard the basic human rights of self-determination, consent to participate in research or unusual clinical activities must be obtained from the prospective subject or his legal representative. Free and informed consent is expected to incorporate the following entities: an explanation of the study, the procedures to be followed, and their purposes; a description of physical risk or discomfort, any invasion of privacy, and any threat to dignity; and the methods used to protect anonymity and to insure confidentiality. The subject needs also to receive a description of any benefits to the subject and/or to the development of new knowledge that potentially might be expected. In instances in which control groups are utilized and therapeutic measures, such as drugs, as withheld, appropriate alternative procedures that might be advantageous for the subject need to be discussed with him

In addition to making available explicit information, an offer to discuss or answer additional questions must be made. The investigator also must inform the subject that he is free to discontinue participation in the activity at any time that he wishes to do so. If subjects are patients of other practitioners, the investigator has an obligation to discuss the proposed study with that individual prior to its inception and to negotiate support for its successful completion.

Subsequent to having all of the above information, the person's consent must be voluntarily given without overt or covert coercion being used and without deception being practiced upon the subject. Should the research design require some degree of concealment of the true purpose or methodology of the study, the design must also provide for subsequent disclosure of the nature of the concealment and the rationale for incorporating secrecy as part of the procedure.

On some occasions, a research design involves procedures or possible outcomes that may impinge upon the rights of someone related to the subject, such as a spouse or parent. In such cases the informed consent of that individual must also be obtained.

The informed consent of parents or legal guardians must be obtained for investigations that involve minors or individuals judged to be legally incompetent to handle their own affairs. In instances in which these subjects have the capacity to comprehend the implications of the proposed activity, they should also be asked to give their consent. In this case, consent supplements rather than supplants that of the parent or other legal agent.

As part of any study protocol, documentation of the procedures to be followed in obtaining informed consent is expected. If written consent is not to be obtained, justification of the omission must be provided. Since the investigator carries the major responsibility for insuring that the rights of the subject are protected, he must throughout the course of the investigation and thereafter scrupulously adhere to the mutual agreement (whether oral or written) contracted with each subject.

Assurance—Institutions and Agencies

There is increasing public support for systematic accountability to insure that unintentional professional and/or investigator bias does not overtly or covertly deny individuals their rights. In almost all circumstances, either the professional nurse or the prospective subject is under the aegis of an institution or agency, and the institution is responsible for establishing and maintaining procedures to safeguard human rights. In most instances, the protective mechanism takes place through a committee judged competent to review projects and other activities that involve human subjects. Membership on the review committee should be representative of all occupational groups (including practicing nurses) whose members are likely to be involved either directly or indirectly in the implementation of the activities or projects undertaken.

In most institutions, the committee is responsible for an initial and continuing review and approval of each activity deemed necessary for review. The review is designed to determine and assure that subject rights have been protected, that the procedures proposed for obtaining informed consent are adequate, that appropriate records are maintained regarding the selection, participation, and protection of subjects, and that circumstances that may or do adversely affect the rights or the welfare of individual subjects are reviewed and acted upon appropriately, In addition, when projects are supported by government funds, the institution must also provide for appropriate professional attention in case the subject suffers physical, psychological, or other injury as a result of participation in the particular activity. In some institutions investigators must also explain how and when identifying data are to be destroyed when the study has been completed.

There are investigational areas in which, by the nature of the data used and the manipulations applied to it, consent by subjects is not required. This ruling would apply to stored data, information, tissue, body fluids, or other materials obtained in the course of routine, professional or clinical observations and activities, and collection does not involve any increased risk to the subject. According to societal values as represented by the federal government, however, use of any of these items for many research, training, and service purposes may present psychological, sociological, or legal risks to the subject or his authorized representative. Determination of whether such risks are involved and whether the use of the materials is within the scope of the original consent is a responsibility of the institution through its established review committee.

In clinical studies that involve hospital or other institutional staff in addition to the research team, special precautions are needed to safeguard the human rights of these employees. If the research design requires actions by persons who are not regular members of the research staff (such as nurses assigned to a clinical unit), steps must be taken to insure that these persons are informed about the procedures and activities expected of them. Responsibility for obtaining informed consent to participate in research belongs to the principal investigator and must not be delegated to regular employees of the institution for the sake of convenience. So that all members of the institutional staff can know that research is in progress, a copy of the patient's (consumer's) signed consent form should be attached as part of that patient's (consumer's) hospital record.

To monitor the utilization of both patients and nursing personnel in research and other special activities, a list of all research projects approved by the institutional review committee must be sent routinely to nursing and other departments that are likely to be involved in the implementation of the studies. Conversely, to safeguard the overutilization of patients and nursing personnel in research and other special projects and to provide a mechanism for approving research and special activities within departments of nursing, organized nursing services have responsibility to develop and enforce written policies and guidelines governing these matters with special attention to protection of the rights of prospective subjects. Guidelines designed to protect human subjects against violation of their rights must incorporate explicit directions for protecting the highly vulnerable individuals who for one or more reasons have difficulty in providing informed consent. High risk individuals include but may not be limited to those who are illiterate, lack command of the English language (or other primary language), do not recognize their right to refuse participation without jeopardizing their care, or for some reason are unable to comprehend instructions or directions.

The institution also has responsibility to formulate mechanisms and procedures for the reporting of events in which human rights are violated. Such mechanisms and procedures need to be brought to the attention of all members of the staff and all consumers of services. The mechanism of reporting should be such that the rights of the person reporting the event also are not violated.

Assurance—Professions

Increased use of hospitals and health care facilities for clinical and other research means that practicing nurses in many institutions are knowingly or unknowingly serving as participants in research designed and implemented by others. Increased educational opportunity for nurses has produced a corps of nurse researchers who are actively engaged in scientific study. Yet stereotyped images of nurses and nursing have in some settings obstructed active participation by nurses on institutional committees for review of research. The profession of nursing through its organization, the American Nurses' Association, has an obligation to publicly support the inclusion of nurses as regular members of the institutional review committees and to make this policy known through written statements of policy.

Because nurses in practice encounter many patients whose rights can unknowingly or inadvertently be violated, the profession of nursing through its national organization carries additional responsibility for the development of written policies and guidelines governing the rights of human subjects to guide nurses at many different levels of practice in formulating policies and procedures pertaining to these matters in their own jurisdictions. The professional nurse's responsibility for protecting the rights of human subjects requires that mechanisms be established whereby violations of rights can be reported and actions taken to countermand the violations. The profession of nursing through its organization at the state level has responsibility to develop mechanisms whereby grievances of nurses may be reported and redressed when these nurses have knowledge of violation of human rights.

PERSONAL RESPONSIBILITY

In order for nursing to fulfill its professional obligations in a rapidly changing society, each nurse must develop an awareness of the issues and a framework for dealing effectively with emerging human rights problems. Ethical issues frequently involve conflicting values, and in many individual cases ethical standards are not specified in sufficient clarity to allow for unambiguous decision-making. As knowledgeable participants in health care practice and research, professional nurses should involve themselves in institutional policy making and review committee activities.

As knowledgeable participants, nurses need also to become informed about various legal parameters affecting practitioner-client relationships. With respect to human rights, legal accountability focuses upon evidence that the professional practitioner or researcher has not failed his/her responsibility by either intentionally or unintentionally withholding relevant information that might have altered the patient or subject's decision. Knowledge about the changing scope of nursing responsibility and the emerging ethical issues affecting all practitioners in health care today is a necessary requirement for professional nursing practice in which accountability for the protection of human rights of consumers is accepted.

BIBLIOGRAPHY

1976 BERGMAN R: Evolving ethical concepts for nursing. INTERNATIONAL NURSING REVIEW 23(4):116-7, Jul-Aug 76, International Council of Nurses.

HUGHES-FORD: The importance of ethics and etiquette to the nursing profession. LAMP, New South Wales Nurses Association 33(1):17-8, Jan 76, Australia.

MURPHY MA; MURPHY J: Making ethical decisions—systematically. NURSING (Jenkintown, Pa.) 6(5):CG 13-4, May 76, USA.

PERRY KL: Accountability: a student's viewpoint. NATIONAL LEAGUE FOR NURSING PUBLICATIONS (16-1621):64-8, 1976, USA.

Editorial: The courage to complain. NURSING MIRROR AND MIDWIVES JOURNAL 142(15):33, 8 Apr 76, England.

Ethics of nursing research. NEW ZEALAND NURSING JOURNAL 69(3):2, Mar 76, New Zealand.

1975 ADOTE AM; BWIRE TL: Ethics and nursing. KENYA NURSING JOURNAL 4(2):14-5, Dec 75, Kenya.

MACKAY RC; SOULE JA: Nurses as investigators: some ethical and legal issues. CANADIAN NURSE 71(9):26-9, Sep 75, Canada.

NORTON D: The research ethic. NURSING TIMES 71(52):2048-9, 25 Dec 75, England.

SWARD KM: The code for nurses: a guide for ethical nursing practice. JOURNAL of the NEW YORK STATE NURSES ASSOCIATION 6(4):25-32, Dec 75, USA.

TAAFFE TC: A concept of professionalism; accountability and responsibility. WORLD OF IRISH NURSING 4(11):1-2, Nov 75, Ireland.

Human rights guidelines for nurses in clinical and other research. No. D-46. AMERICAN NURSES ASSOCIATION PUBLICATION (D-46):1-11, Jul 75, USA.

Bibliography obtained from the World Health Organization Medline Centre, Office of Library and Health Literature Services, Geneva, Switzerland. Includes articles published in English 1971-76.

1974 ALLEN M: Ethics of nursing practice. CANADIAN NURSE 70(2):22-3, Feb 74, Canada.

CARNEGIE ME: The patient's bill of rights and the nurse. NURSING CLINICS OF NORTH AMERICA 9(3):557-62, Sept 74, USA.

CIPRIANO SILVA M: Science, ethics and nursing. AMERICAN JOURNAL OF NURSING 74(11):2004-7, Nov 74, USA.

CREIGHTON H: Moral and legal issues—nursing judgments. No. 16-1551. NATIONAL LEAGUE FOR NURSING PUBLICATIONS (16-1551):22, May 74, USA.

DICKENS BM: The 'conscience clause' and the law on abortion. NURSING TIMES 70(25):968-9, 20 Jun 74, England.

IU S: President's address at International Nurses Day celebration. 7th May, 1947, City Hall Theatre. HONG KONG NURSING JOURNAL (17):6-9, Nov 74, Hong Kong.

JEGEDE: Nurses code of ethics and legal implications in nursing practice. NIGERIAN NURSE 6(3):34-41, Jul-Sep 74, Nigeria.

LAMERTON R: Symposium: care of the dying; ethical questions in the care of the dying. NURSING MIRROR and MIDWIVES JOURNAL 139(15):61-3, 10 Oct 74, England.

PELLS J: Prolonging life. 4. Nurse's burden, doctor's decision. NURSING TIMES 70(11):393-4, 14 Mar 74, England.

SWABY G: What's in the nurses' new code? JAMAICAN NURSE 14(3):21-2, Dec 74, Jamaica.

Code of ethics as applied to nursing. INTERNATIONAL NURSING REVIEW 21(3-4):103-4, May-Aug 74, International Council of Nurses.

Editorial: The ridiculous trump. AUSTRALIAN NURSES' JOURNAL 3(9):5, Apr 74, Australia.

Nursing ethics; the admirable professional standards of nurses: a survey report. Part 2. Honesty, confidentiality, termination of life, and other decisions in nursing. NURSING (Jenkintown, Pa.) 4(10):56-66, Oct 74, USA.

Quandary: accepting gifts. NURSING TIMES 70(3):72, 17 Jan 74, England.

1973 BAKER E: On Teaching ethics to nurses. NURSING TIMES, England, 69:683-4, 24 May 73.

BERGMAN R: Translating a nursing belief into nursing practice. AUSTRALASIAN NURSING JOURNAL 2:9, Jul 73.

BERGMAN R: Ethics—Concept and practice. INTERNATIONAL NURSING REVIEW, ICN Switzerland 20:140-1, Sep-Oct 73.
CREIGHTON H: Law for the nurse-supervisor. ICN's new code for nurses. SUPERVISOR NURSE, USA. 4:13-5, Sep 73.
FOUGERAT AJ: Introduction to code of ethics for nurses. IRISH NURSING NEWS 152:11-2, Spring 73.
FOUGERAT AJ: Nurse of tomorrow, will you still be master of your conscience. IRISH NURSING NEWS 152:21-3, Spring 73.
FOUGERAT AJ: Nurses of tomorrow, will you still be master of your conscience. IRISH NURSING NEWS 153:19-24, Summer 73.
HARRIS CH: Some ethical and legal considerations in neonatal intensive care. NURSING CLINICS OF NORTH AMERICA, USA 8:521-31, Sep 73.
HORTON L: What will happen to Mr. Lang. CANADIAN NURSE 69:39-40, May 73.
KELLY DN: The code of ethics. SUPERVISOR NURSE, USA 4:7, Sep 73.
McPHERSON D: Problems of professionalism with particular reference to nursing. JAMAICAN NURSE 13:26-7, Aug-Sep 73.
ROSE V: Careless talk can cause misery. NURSING MIRROR and MIDWIVES JOURNAL, England 136:14, 5 Jan 73.
SCHORR TM: Magna Carta for nurses everywhere. AMERICAN JOURNAL OF NURSING 73:1329, Aug 73.
SCHRADER ES: OR nurses face decision in abortion procedures. AORN JOURNAL, USA. 17:13-6, May 73.
SMART M: Who is man. NEW ZEALAND NURSING JOURNAL. 66:22-4, May 73.
TYRER LB, GRANZIG WA: The new morality, ethics, and nursing. JOURNAL OF OBSTETRIC, GYNECOLOGIC AND NEONATAL NURSING, USA. 2:54-5, Sep-Oct 73.
Code of ethics for nurses. IRISH NURSING NEWS 152:13-4, Spring 73.
ICN nurses' code. AUSTRALIAN NURSES' JOURNAL 3:17, Oct 73.
Quandary hidden wealth. NURSING TIMES, England 69:1717, 20 Dec 73.

1972 BERGER AL: What would you do...PENNSYLVANIA NURSE USA 17:7, Mar 72.

CROSS Y: Nursing the cruel. NURSING MIRROR and MIDWIVES JOURNAL, England 134:9-12, 17 Mar 72.
FLAHERTY J: The present of today was the future of yesterday. RNAO NEWS, Canada 28:11-3, May-Jun 72.
FOUGERAT AJ: Nurse of tomorrow, will you still be master of your conscience. IRISH NURSING NEWS 23-7, Winter 72.
JUPP V: Professionalization and new forms of nursing education. INTERNATIONAL JOURNAL OF NURSING STUDIES, England 19:19-25, Mar 72.
SCHORR TM: Issues of conscience. AMERICAN JOURNAL OF NURSING 72:61, Jan 72.
VENTER ME: Discussion of the Nursing Act No. 69 of 1957 as amended by the Nursing Amendment Act No. 50 of 1972 and matters relating to it. SOUTH AFRICAN NURSING JOURNAL 39:22-8, Oct 72.
WHINCUP MH: Confidentiality and the law. OCCUPATIONAL HEALTH, England 24:352-3, Oct 72.
Ethics of nursing research. CANADIAN NURSE 68:23-5, Sep 72.
King's Fund transatlantic nursing seminar. NURSING TIMES, England 68:149-52, 21 Sep 72.

1971 CROSS Y, MACKENZIE N: Life and living it. NURSING MIRROR and MIDWIVES JOURNAL, England 133:49-51, 15 Oct 71.
GODFREY J: The (multiple) meaning of values. AUSTRALIAN NURSES JOURNAL 1:32-4, Jul 71.
GOLUB S, REZNIKOFF M: Attitudes toward death. A comparison of nursing students and graduate nurses. NURSING RESEARCH, USA 20:503-8, Nov-Dec 71.
LIPMAN M: When should a nurse blow the whistle. R.N., USA 34:50-2, Oct 71.
MATHEW G: Therapeutic abortion. Nurses' involvement and moral grounds. NURSING JOURNAL OF INDIA 62:305-6, Sep 71.